MOMENTS
that matter

MOMENTS
that
matter

DEFINING MOMENTS THAT
shifted everything

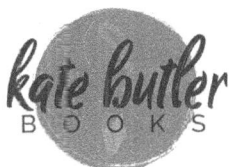

kate butler
B O O K S

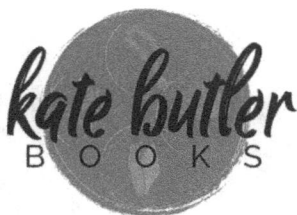

Published by Kate Butler Books

Cover and interior design by Melissa Williams Design

ISBN: 978-1-962407-33-5

table of contents

Featuring Author

Eichelle V. Thompson

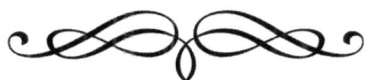

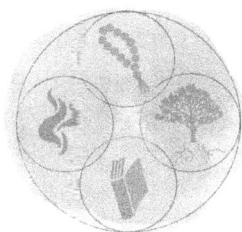

GREATNESS IN THE MOMENT

Eichelle V. Thompson

In the 2019 NBA Eastern Conference Semifinals, I watched Toronto Raptors' forward Kawhi Leonard hit the final two-point shot from the far-right corner. The ball bobbled four times—four times—before dropping in at the buzzer to win game seven of their playoff series against the Sixers.

Leonard had been great all season and great during the playoff series. He had done his job every minute of every quarter of every game—all season long. But, when game seven was on the line to advance his team and he got the ball, it wasn't enough that he had been great in any other game. He needed to be great in that moment.

He probably wasn't thinking of past failures or past successes, like so many of us do. He just needed to get the job done at that moment. It was seconds, fractions of seconds, that played out on the court. The world watched as the sum of a player's career, with the team on his back, came down to one shot. That's a lot of pressure. In life, most of us hope never to be in that position. Even Leonard, crouched low in the corner waiting for the ball to drop, must have wondered in the moment: Will I be great enough?

Throughout the series, both teams battled back and forth,

fighting for every foul, every free throw, every possession, neither acquiescing even as it became a one-point game in the last four seconds. But, in those last moments, it wasn't the team that got the ball, it was a single player: Leonard.

We know that a game is won or lost by the team. Yet, that win-lose binary sits upon a fulcrum, a point that can feel very singular. No matter what game is being played, winning is a process that depends upon successful moments.

Theodore Roosevelt once said, "The credit belongs to the man who is actually in the arena, the one who is daring greatly."[1] Some might say Roosevelt was giving credit to the competitors like Leonard, the fighters who have evaluated their opponent and enter the arena to win. Certainly, this competitor is "daring greatly."

What if Roosevelt wasn't paying homage to the competition? What if he was turning the spotlight inward to examine the very act of stepping into the arena?

After all, there is a moment when we make the choice not to just step in, but to step in in spite of our deficits. Wasn't Roosevelt giving credit to the single moment when we ignore the critics both outside and within ourselves and step into the arena anyway? Surely, even Leonard had his doubts.

Both Roosevelt and Leonard highlight the decision to step into the arena at all. They reveal the courage it takes to be willing to discover our limits, to trust that the past is enough to deliver the future. In an arena as big and public as the NBA Semifinals, that takes a lot of courage. Roosevelt validates it. He gives intrinsic value to the struggle and credit to the believers who enter any arena knowing they may lose but believing they can win. They are the players, the parents, the creators, the entrepreneurs.

In fact, each moment is at once the win, the loss, and the learning. Roosevelt dares us to be great in every single one of them, so we have a foundation to land upon when we fall. He

1 "The Man in the Arena," Theodore Roosevelt Center, Dickinson State University, accessed July 26, 2023, https://www.theodorerooseveltcenter. org/Learn-About-TR/TR-Encyclopedia/Culture-and-Society/Man-in-the-Arena.aspx

acknowledges that there is a difference between greatness and being the greatest and that the former is the better to be.

Most of us will never be NBA-level athletes like Leonard or CEOs of multimillion-dollar international businesses. We won't be widely influential or even "influencers." But we will be called upon to be great.

I grew up in the '60s hearing the messages of feminists. Girls can do anything boys can do, they said. I believed it. My tomboy child-self tested the theory, desperately wanting to be great at something. Anything. I entered many arenas that were then dominated by boys. I climbed trees, played soccer and softball. I rode a mini-bike and learned to snowboard. As an adult, I fought against unnecessary dress codes that left me and my female colleagues wearing skirts in winter. Throughout my life, I found the courage to challenge myself, my own beliefs and fears, and those of others.

Sometimes, life felt tough and heavy. Big decisions, tough challenges, fearful moments. If the critic in me showed up at the arena door, bravery waned and I felt my big dreams slipping away.

Then, the optimist in me would regroup, evaluate, and try again from a smaller arena. Over time, the size of the arena ceased to matter. Winning and losing became fluid, more adjectives than conclusions, and I began to see the intrinsic value of not only the struggle, but also the moment I chose to take it on, in spite of.

Time and time again, I found my limits, my resilience and my greatness.

And so, when I see players like Leonard entering the arena, I cheer and support them because I know that regardless of the outcome of the game, it's not about what you take away from the experience—the trophy or the title—it's what you leave on the court or the field or the ring or the track or the office or in the home that matters. It's about knowing you were all in. You pulled out all the stops when you had to. You tried harder when you felt there was nothing left to give. You pushed past the adversity, crushed the naysayers, dominated your own inner doubt, and left yourself no discussion points on whether you could have or should have. Those points are mute because you played the moments right. And you played them in the moment.

But first, you stepped into the arena, in spite of. That's something of courage.

So, when the NBA series was on the line and Leonard got the ball, we inhaled because he held that ball for all of us. We watched as he fought his way to the right corner. The crowd stood. We held our collective breath as the ball left Leonard's fingertips with .3 seconds on the clock. The players on both teams froze, eyes wide and mouths open, tracking the ball as it arced from the corner to the rim with precision. Leonard crouched as time stretched. The silence was broken by the sound of the ball as, like a judge's mallet, it hit the rim those four times—clunk, clunk, clunk, clunk.

We waited to see if Leonard would be great—not the whole game or the whole series or the whole season. We waited to see if Leonard was going to be great in that single moment. As soon as the ball dropped past the rim, we knew he was.

The question is, if the ball would have dropped out, would Leonard have still been great?

The answer is yes.

Because greatness is not about being the greatest. Greatness, rather, is defined by what you bring to the struggle, how you play out the moments, especially the one where you decide to enter the arena.

Go and be great. This moment is yours.

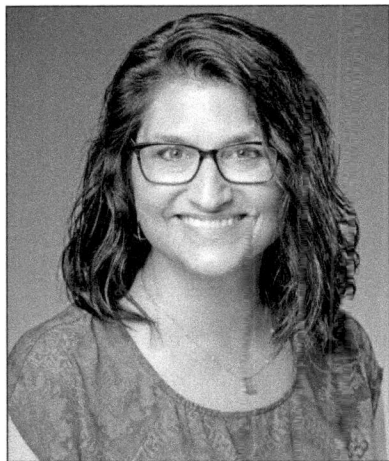

ABOUT EICHELLE V. THOMPSON

Eichelle is a writer and artist, with a thirty-two-year professional background in various areas of marketing. She has enjoyed working in a wide range of industries including visual arts, communications, higher education, and construction. She holds a Bachelor of Arts degree in journalism/mass communications from the University of Wisconsin—Milwaukee and a Master of Arts degree in creative writing from Mount Mary University.

Based just outside of Milwaukee, Wisconsin, Eichelle draws creative inspiration from her experiences as a professional and from her roles as first-born, first-generation American, sister, wife, mother, grandmother, and friend.

In this Moments That Matter collaboration, Eichelle examines the self-doubt, fear, and social pressures we experience throughout our lives. She challenges our definition of "greatness" and asks: who is the keeper of the label?

To learn more about Eichelle and her work, visit:

www.eichelle.com

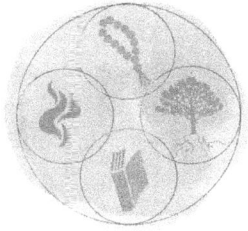

FOREWORD

Patty Aubery

Life has a way of surprising us, doesn't it? It can lift us to exhilarating heights, cradle us in moments of bliss, and yet, in an instant, it can snatch it all away, leaving us grappling with a sense of profound loss. These are the moments that shake us to our core, revealing the fragile nature of our existence and reminding us of the urgency to embrace every precious second we have.

I still remember the day when my world tilted on its axis. It was a time of darkness a time when my heart became heavy with grief and my spirit yearned for solace. My mother, my pillar of strength, had been diagnosed with breast cancer, a relentless adversary that threatened to steal her away from us. As her body weakened, her spirit grew stronger, and she taught me one of the most valuable lessons life has ever bestowed upon me.

In the quiet moments we shared, she looked into my eyes, her voice filled with love and determination. "Promise me," she whispered, "promise me that you will not hide. Embrace life in all its rawness, in all its vulnerability. Promise me that you will seize every moment, for it is in those moments that life's true magic resides."

Those words pierced my heart, etching themselves deep into

my being. They became my compass, guiding me through the labyrinth of grief, and inspiring me to make the most of the time I have been granted. It is this personal journey, forged through loss and fueled by an unwavering love, that led me to share my story within the pages of this book.

As you embark on this reading journey, I invite you to connect with the universal truths that bind us all together. Life's moments—both the magnificent and the devastating—have a way of shaping us, transforming us into the individuals we are meant to become. In the midst of heartache, we discover our resilience, our capacity for compassion, and our unwavering spirit. And in the moments of pure joy, we uncover the essence of what it means to truly live.

This book is not just about my story; it is about our shared humanity. It is an invitation to reflect upon your own journey, the pivotal moments that have marked your path, and the legacy you are creating through the choices you make. It is a reminder that life's fragility is a gift—an urgent call to embrace the fleeting nature of our existence, to hold close those we cherish, and to honor the moments that touch our souls.

As you read these pages, allow yourself to be fully present. Let the stories shared here stir something within you, perhaps awakening dormant dreams or reminding you of the value of the relationships that enrich your life. May you find solace, inspiration, and a renewed commitment to live authentically, cherishing each moment as the precious gift that it is.

In life, even in the difficult moments, we have a choice—to retreat and hide from life's uncertainties, or to step boldly into the world, allowing our hearts to remain open to all that it offers. It is my deepest desire that this book serves as a gentle reminder to seize every opportunity, to celebrate the beauty of each fleeting moment, and to embrace the fragility of life with courage and grace.

Dear reader, as you embark on this profound exploration of

life's fleeting moments, I extend my hand to you, knowing that within the pages of this book, we share a common thread of resilience, loss, and the unwavering pursuit of meaning. Together, let us walk this path, honoring the memories that have shaped us and the moments that continue to shape us still. In our shared experiences, may we find solace connection, and the inspiration to embrace life with unwavering courage and an unyielding appreciation for the precious moments that make up our existence.

With heartfelt gratitude,

Patty Aubery

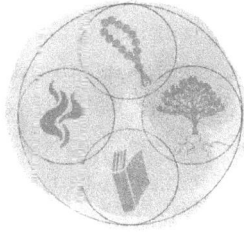

INTRODUCTION
FROM THE INSPIRED IMPACT
SERIES CREATOR

Kate Butler, CPSC

Life is a magnificent tapestry woven with countless moments, each holding the potential to shape our journey. From the smallest interactions to the grandest milestones, every moment we experience plays a vital role in our personal growth and the unfolding of our unique purpose. In this chapter, we will delve into the profound significance of embracing each moment along the way, recognizing that life's purpose is intricately intertwined with continuous growth. Together, let us explore the profound truth that every moment matters.

Life is a journey of growth, an ever-unfolding path. It is not a stagnant destination but a dynamic journey that unfolds with every passing moment. It is a series of interconnected steps that propel us forward, urging us to learn, evolve, and expand our horizons. We must recognize that growth is the very essence of our existence and that we are never truly done growing. By embracing this truth, we unlock the potential for profound transformation in every aspect of our lives.

Life's journey is a dance between discovery and becoming. We embark on this path as curious beings, eager to explore the vast landscape of human experience. As we take steps forward, we encounter challenges, triumphs, and moments of profound insight. Each experience shapes us, molding us into more resilient, compassionate, and self-aware individuals.

Embracing the process is part of the fun! Life's purpose lies not in reaching a final destination but in embracing the process of becoming. Each moment serves as a stepping-stone, leading us toward our true potential. It is through the cumulative effect of these moments, the lessons learned, and the experiences gained, that we discover our purpose and shape our unique identity. By embracing the journey and allowing ourselves to be present in each moment, we open ourselves up to the infinite possibilities that await us.

Embracing the process requires a shift in perspective. It invites us to release the pressure of external expectations and the benchmarks of our paradigms. Instead, we focus on the internal growth and personal evolution that occurs with each step we take. We learn to honor the twists and turns of our journey, appreciating the detours and the moments of uncertainty as opportunities for growth and self-discovery.

There is a power of presence in our mindful awareness. To fully embrace each moment, we must cultivate a state of mindful awareness. By grounding ourselves in the present, we become attuned to the richness and depth of our experiences. Mindfulness allows us to engage with life wholeheartedly, free from the constraints of past regrets or future anxieties. Through this practice, we learn to appreciate the beauty and significance of even the simplest moments, finding joy and meaning in the here and now.

Practicing mindfulness involves directing our attention to the present moment with non-judgmental awareness. We cultivate a deep connection with our thoughts, emotions, and physical sensations, anchoring ourselves in the present. This heightened awareness allows us to fully immerse ourselves in the experiences that unfold before us, savoring the textures, colors, and nuances of life. By embracing the power of presence, we unlock the transformative potential of every moment.

We must find purpose in the ordinary. Moments that matter are not confined to grand achievements or monumental events. They also exist in the everyday occurrences, the seemingly mundane interactions, and the quiet, introspective moments. By recognizing the inherent value in each experience, we elevate the ordinary to the extraordinary. We discover that our purpose is not solely tied to extraordinary acts but is deeply rooted in the way we show up in every moment, infusing it with love, compassion, and authenticity.

Finding purpose in the ordinary requires a shift in perception. It is a practice of presence, allowing us to view the world through a lens of wonder and gratitude. When we open ourselves to the beauty of simplicity, we unlock a profound appreciation for life's smallest details. The smile exchanged with a stranger, the warmth of a cup of tea on a chilly morning, or the quiet moments of solitude become opportunities to connect, reflect, and grow.

The ripple effect is the most powerful part. Embracing every moment as an opportunity for growth has a profound impact on our own personal development. As we seize each moment with intention and purpose, we cultivate resilience, adaptability, and self-awareness. We learn from our mistakes, celebrate our successes, and continually refine our understanding of who we are and what we are capable of. Each moment becomes a catalyst for personal transformation, propelling us closer to our fullest potential.

When we embrace the moments that matter, we embark on a profound journey of self-discovery. We recognize that growth requires vulnerability and a willingness to step out of our comfort zones. By embracing challenges and the discomfort that accompanies growth, we unlock our true potential. We discover the depths of our strength, the expansiveness of our hearts, and the vastness of our capabilities.

The significance of each moment extends beyond ourselves. Our actions, words, and presence have the power to ripple out and touch the lives of others. When we embrace the moments that matter, we become agents of positive change, inspiring and uplifting those around us. By fostering authentic connections and showing up fully in our interactions, we create a ripple effect of growth, love, and empowerment that reverberates far beyond the immediate moment.

Our interactions with others hold the potential to be transformative. By embracing moments of connection, we can uplift and support those we encounter. A kind word, a listening ear, or a gesture of empathy can have a profound impact on someone's life. When we recognize the interconnectedness of our experiences, we understand that our growth and the growth of others are intimately intertwined. Each moment becomes an opportunity to make a difference, to leave a positive imprint on the lives of those we encounter.

In the grand tapestry of life, each moment is a thread that weaves together our journey of growth and purpose. By recognizing that our life's purpose is intricately tied to continuous growth, we unlock the transformative power inherent in every experience. Embracing the moments that matter means embracing the present, recognizing that even the simplest interaction holds the potential for profound impact. As we embark on this journey of self-discovery and personal evolution, let us embrace each moment with an open heart and an open mind, knowing that our purpose lies in the unwavering commitment to growth and the understanding that every moment matters.

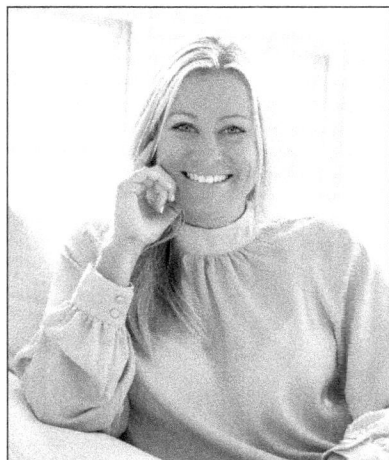

ABOUT KATE BUTLER, CPSC

Kate Butler is a #1 International Best-selling and Award-winning author and speaker. As a CPSC, Certified Professional Success Coach, she offers clients dynamic programs to help them reach their ultimate potential and live out their dreams. She does this through mindset, success, and book publishing programs. Kate is also the creator of the Inspired Impact Book Series, which has published twelve titles.

Kate received her double major degree in Mass Communications and Interpersonal Communication Studies from Towson University in Maryland. After ten years in the corporate world, Kate decided it was time to fulfill her true passion; she studied business at Wharton School of Business at The University of Pennsylvania and received her certificate in Entrepreneur Acceleration.

Kate now brings her expertise to mainstream media where she has been featured as the Mindset and Publishing expert on Fox 29, Good Day Philadelphia, HBO, in the Huffington Post, and on various other television, news, and radio platforms.

To learn more about becoming an author in the Inspired Impact Book Series, or to learn how to work with Kate directly on achieving your goals or publishing your book (including children's books), visit her website at www.katebutlerbooks.com. Kate would love to connect with you!

To Connect with Kate:

Facebook: @katebutlerbooks
Instagram: @katebutlerbooks
Website: www.katebutlerbooks.com

Bella Butler
started writing books at
the age of 5 and became a
#1 Best-selling Author with her debut
children's book, *More Than Magic*. At age
9 she became a #1 International Best-selling
Author with her second book, *Believe Big*.
Ever since then, she has dreamed of bringing her
writing to the adult space. Bella has diligently
worked on her writing to refine her craft, with the
dream of her non-fiction work being published
one day. What will unfold next *is* what Bella
calls *her* Moment That Matters…her dream
of being published in this space, coming
true. Thank you all for being a part
of this special moment.
To the unfolding…

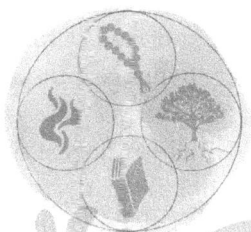

A Year to Remember

Bella Butler

The first day of school isn't everyone's favorite, especially when you're going to a new school. My first day of seventh grade was different from any other first day of school, and it wasn't because I felt like the new kid (I was used to it by now). It was because *nobody* talked to me. I was used to introducing myself to others, but there wasn't any time for that. When we were packing up to go home, one girl came over and introduced herself. She didn't have to, but she did. That one act of kindness made my day.

A few days later, I went to my seat in English class. Another girl sat next to me. I had only talked to one person so far this year, and I was trying to change that. But before I could, the teacher called for our attention. She handed out textbooks and workbooks, and once she was done, she asked everyone to take out a piece of paper. As I dug through my bag, the girl next to me already had two sheets of paper out. When she offered one to me, I smiled and accepted. Now, I had two friends.

As the month of September went on, I was getting acclimated to my new school. I even ran for our student council's treasurer.

We had to write a speech and read it for the *whole school.* Many people saw this as another challenge, but I saw it as a bonus! People made flyers and signs trying to get votes, and I really wanted to do that too, however I still didn't have a speech. The night before it was due, I wrote and practiced my speech. The next day the candidates for student council lined up across the stage. I was running for treasurer against one other kid, but he was in eighth grade and had been at the school for years. I was brand new, and it was only September, so not many people knew me. After we gave our speeches, the students voted. It took a few days, but the results were in. They announced the new members of the student council over the loudspeaker, so the whole school could hear it. *"And our new treasurer is . . . Bella Butler!"* I screamed in front of my whole class! I couldn't believe it! I was the newest member of the student council.

The year continued, and there weren't many events going on at school, besides the build up to winter break. Everyone was getting bored of school, but I was getting bored at school. The curriculum was easier than what I was hoping for when we joined the school, and I even wanted to switch schools, but I didn't. I'm very grateful for that. I continued to work hard and achieve as much as possible. Winter break kept me going because I would *finally* have a break from the drama, the fights, and the boredom of school. My math teacher was super nice, but I don't think he *quite* understood me. He grouped me with all of the other kids in the advanced math class (like any other teacher would) and he would teach the same lesson to all of us. While some kids needed extra help, my friend from English class and I excelled in this class. We both induced many emails from our parents to our teacher. He attempted to refine his lessons, but we both were very intellectual. When he did evolve the curriculum, I was engaged in it for the rest of the year.

Our cheer team had our first competition when we got back from winter break. All of us were thrilled, and when we were at the competition, our expectations were surpassed. Even though we didn't get first place, we were all so proud of ourselves! This moment was a great way to resume the school year. Our team still had some impediments, but we overcame them and had an epic cheer season!!!

As the year went on, the teachers started to improve their lessons for some other students and me. It was harder to pass each test and quiz, and that was a good thing. I enjoyed school more and more. After auditioning for our school play, I got a lead role! I even had my own song. For some reason I reluctantly joined the track team, but after the first practice, I'm so glad I did. These were the highlights of my school year. I was at rehearsals, practices, and track meets almost every single day of the week, and I loved every moment of it. I made many friends because of both activities, and I had the most fun ever. Track meets were all day, but my friends and I got to hang out, and outshine our previous records. At play rehearsals, I sang my heart out, and recited every line from memory after a few short weeks. We had three performances of our play, plus numerous track meets. In fact, we had a track meet the same night as our final performance. I ran hard that day and was exhausted (and sunburnt) after, but my final performance was 100% my best effort. I even sang afterwards at the restaurant where we ate. People called me by my stage name all around school, and people from the track team still hung out and exchanged inside jokes. The season might have been over, but the memories we made were lifelong.

At the end of the year, when I was signing yearbooks, I would write a whole paragraph in everyone's yearbooks about all of the amazing memories we made. When I was writing about all of these moments, I realized how much each one mattered to me. At some points throughout the school year I felt like a prisoner, but I also had many more memories where I was as free as an eagle. This school year had its ups and downs from unexpected fights and overwhelming drama to the privilege of getting a lead role in the play, being the student council treasurer, racing around the track with friends, and being co-captain of the school cheer team. Seventh grade was a year to remember, and I made so many friends and memories. This year will have a lasting impact on the rest of my life, and I'm so grateful that I was able to achieve all of the incredible things I've done as a middle schooler. Even with high school looming ahead, I will always remember these moments that (no matter how small) mattered.

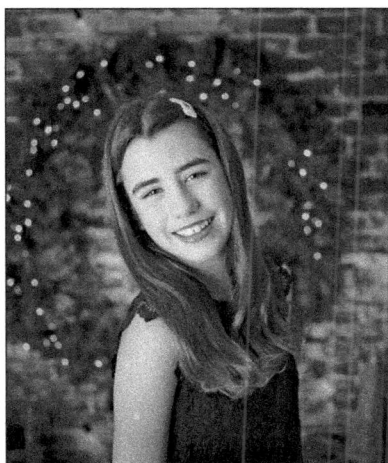

ABOUT BELLA BUTLER

Bella Butler is 13 years old and entering eighth grade. She is a two-time #1 best-selling author who loves to read and write whenever possible.

Bella travels the globe as an inspirational speaker and author. Her goal is to connect with as many children as possible to teach them the power of their thoughts in a way children can understand and from someone they can relate to! Bella's unique teachings have been brought all over the United States, Canada, Grenada, Ireland, Italy, and France. Bella has an exquisite way of connecting with all children, in a way that only she can, with her generous spirit and gracious heart. She would love to come to your school, group, community or company to deliver a one-of-kind inspirational keynote or facilitate an experiential author reading. Bella is a true professional and is ready to show up, inspire, and leave the audience with life changing perspectives and tools. Bella's work inspires and transforms children and adults alike! She will come to you, wherever you are in the world! To book Bella, simply reach out to support@katebutlerbooks.com.

When Bella isn't with her books, she is riding horses, volunteering at horse farms, singing, playing piano, or traveling. She believes that all things are possible if you are willing to dream them and is always conquering her own aspirations. You can find her two #1 best-selling books, *More Than Magic* and *Believe Big* on Amazon.com, Barnes & Noble.com and Target.com. She was thrilled to write a chapter in *Moments That Matter*!

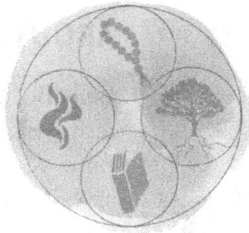

CHASING PRETTY:
THE DAY THE FAT LADY STOPPED SINGING

Erin Saxton

Do you hear that? In the silence of you reading this, if you listen closely, you will hear the buzzing of my procrastination. At present, I am delayed in writing this piece because I have been telling myself I have been 'mulling over' exactly what I want to say. So I am officially calling BS on myself and just chalking it up to the fact that I am nervous to write down what I know I "should" say. Side-note: Rarely do I say "should" to myself and never say "should" to anyone else. A teacher once taught me that saying "should" to anyone is an absolute insult to them, and one's opinion of what someone else "should" do is beyond anyone but that person's own judgment, no one else's. An extreme lesson taught, and while I take it with a grain of salt, I do try to not use that word often, though something tells me it will be used a few times in this text. So what is the real reason behind today's procrastination? The simple answer is I was on autopilot, which is the cousin to procrastination, but we will get to that topic in a bit. The deeper answer is fear.

Now, with a few clicks of my keyboard I am ready to hurdle over that feeling of fear and will write this with the best of intentions of having you get to know me, and in reading my story maybe get a glimpse into my life so you will then realize you are not the only one who may struggle with - anything.

Two years ago I experienced this mack daddy of a moment. The big message in that moment was that I was telling myself that I wanted my life a certain way, but would rely on the excuses as to why they were not coming to fruition when I would put my psyche on AUTOPILOT.

That got me thinking, what else do I do on autopilot? When I really sat with that question I realized I do A LOT on autopilot. I realized that the only two things I rarely have on autopilot is when I am working on my business and parenting my son Erik. Scratch that, I promised to stay transparent. I am positive there are times that I go on autopilot even with my business. Autopilot, I am quickly learning, tricks me into thinking it protects me, but it actually does the opposite. Autopilot did not block me from disappointment, or mend my shattered heart or keep me company when I was lonely. Instead, autopilot told me I needed to snack, have a decadent meal, buy new clothes, order cookware for my kitchen, you get the idea. This had to stop, I had to get to the bottom of this so I forced myself to sit in the uncomfortable feeling of making a list of what I was doing without really "thinking". The list was long. Extremely long.

After I completed the list, I came away with this bonked-over-the-head moment of absolute TRUTH. Living life, or avoiding being present while living life wreaked havoc on me. More importantly, when I was not aware I was on autopilot yucky stuff crept up on me. I was oblivious to it happening and the result was I felt as if I woke up one day and suddenly my jeans didn't fit, my relationship with my partner was dull and I felt disconnected from him, I signed up for Apps that I never even opened, and discovered my big accomplishment of the day was that I achieved a really high level of Fish Kingdom (kind of like Candy Crush but with fish bowls). I felt exhausted like I had been treading water for years, but frankly did not remember even jumping into the swimming pool. What I discovered is that life will distract me if I let it. I also learned that I love to follow the bright shiny objects and bouncy balls and while that is fun, I can get off course. WHAT DO YOU DO WHILE YOU ARE ON AUTOPILOT? I will say this: chances are you are on autopilot if you are overeating, you have been perpetually losing and gaining the same 15 or more pounds year after year, you are potentially having sex with the wrong people, you are spending money on stuff you don't need and likely you could also be in the wrong job/career.

I have painfully discovered that life is a game and there is a wizard behind the curtain pushing buttons to zing me. Sometimes life zings with terrific events (that is when I would fool myself, thinking that I had my life together and all figured out) and other times the zings are painful, which then leaves me thinking situations were worse than they really were. I needed to figure out what I was doing while I was dealing with all of the zings, even the good ones. So I sat in pain, disgust, shame and most importantly, I refused to go on autopilot.

I then realized that all the moments that I was experiencing while I was on autopilot were THE MOMENTS THAT MATTERED THE MOST.

Why Chasing Pretty? For me, I thought I was negatively getting "zinged' left and right because I did not look a certain way. I always thought if someone was fit and thin they had their act together, after all they were able to obtain a body shape that I had aspired to have but always seemed to be out of reach. After all, being thin was the only thing if I really set my mind to do that still escaped me. Thin and fit people must know something that I do not know. I found that intriguing. Intriguing to me is "pretty". Anyone who seems to have it all put together in my opinion is "pretty". They could have a face only their mom would love, but to me, if they were thin, fit and seemingly successful I thought they were "pretty". Consciously I did not realize I was processing any of this like that of course, but in one of my "moments" when I refused to go on autopilot I came upon this realization.

Upon that realization I then dug deeper. What I came to realize was that I did not actually like who I was very much and I was sabotaging myself. Here I am truly thinking I was living my best life and in many cases I was/am truly blessed. But like our friend Eeyore, I was wondering why I was not accomplishing things that I told myself I really wanted: a healthy and fit body, a loving romantic relationship and doing more on camera work etc. Unlike Eeyore, I was genuinely happy for the successes and wins of those I was scrolling by on social media, though if I am staying transparent it did make me wonder, "why not me?" I knew I never wanted to be an onlooker, and I absolutely never want to be envious of others' successes or body shape. People who judge and are jealous of the joy everyone else experiences are likely the ones who avoid looking in the mirror. What those people fail to do is sit down with themselves to figure out why things they say they want are not going their way. And that is what I knew I had to do myself.

So began 2 solid years of looking inward. Along the way I consulted experts, doctors, scientists and psychics on various topics to help me peel back what was what. I began exercising with a trainer, meditated more, took up tennis, and created a plan to shed weight. All along staying "present". If I got hungry I analyzed why I was hungry before taking a bite. If I wanted to cancel a session with my trainer I analyzed that too. Once I began to really lose significant weight I thought I had broken the chain of living on autopilot, and then life threw a zing at me. My neighbor jokingly texted me to say that "the UPS driver must know the way to drive to your house in his sleep by now because he drops off something every other day!" I replied back with a smiley face emoji and knowing her good nature just chalked it up to her humor. Later that day I noticed a package on my porch, the day after that there was a mound of boxes. The next day 2 more boxes arrived. Ah, I then realized, I did not fix anything - I just replaced food with online shopping. Ugh! So I began to unwind that mindless habit again. The result? I am more aware than ever before, but the wicked autopilot is always around the corner. I realized I was binge watching shows one weekend. I mean who could blame me, I am not snacking all that much and I am not ordering excessively from Amazon, so what is a girl to do, right?!! So I shut off the TV and asked myself the following questions: Do I really want what I am saying I am wishing for? What am I in the back of my mind trying to process while I am zoning out on this TV show? What is really going on here? I promised myself if I could figure it out, then I could go back to watching the show. Sometimes the answers would come quickly, other times it took awhile. Either way, I was off autopilot.

My take away from these unaware moments is that I am always trying to either bury what I refuse to deal with or I am avoiding coming to the conclusion about a decision because it may cause conflict or even worse hurt feelings. Now that I know that I no longer need to excessively eat, shop or binge watch TV. What I DO need to do is be aware and face what I am dealing with head on. I will still find myself on autopilot of course, we all will from time to time, but my goal is to not stay in that state of denial for long periods of time.

The best outcome for me getting off autopilot is not not being thin, or having an amazing relationship with the most amazing man or the fact that my credit card number is not being used as much online anymore. The best outcome is that I no longer daydream about how my life "could be", I now realize that I don't have to chase anything because what I need in order to go after the life I want has been inside me all along.

I guarantee that YOU are enough, too. Sit by yourself and think. Ask yourself different questions. Set a random alarm to ring at an odd time of day just to make sure you are not on autopilot somehow. As long as you do not get in your own way, you can accomplish anything.

Whatever you are chasing, stop running, what you need to win is already within you too.

YOU ARE PRETTY.

ABOUT ERIN SAXTON

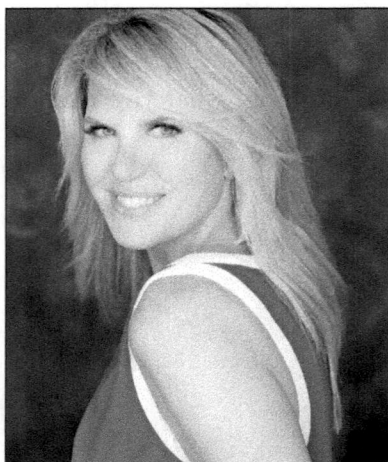

For nearly 20 years, Erin Saxton has been asking the right questions and getting in-depth, meaningful answers. She has conducted thousands of interviews with guests, clients to get to the heart of anyone's story. As powerhouse television producer and protege of Barbara Walters, Erin has received several Emmy nominations for her work with nationally syndicated television shows such as the Barbara Walters Specials, The Rosie O'Donnell Show, Good Morning America and The View. Through that extensive experience, she carved a niche for consulting on and executing effective PR and Marketing campaigns. On leaving The View, Saxton launched her own marketing agency, Erin led the national media strategy for notables like Jack Canfield, who at last count has sold 500 million books. Her knowledge extends across B2B and B2C markets, and she is actively involved in associations and events, delivering keynote addresses as an expert in her field to business audiences around the country. As an expert in the field of Public Relations, Erin is known to have a proven track record of delivering repeated successes to her clients, whether small-to-medium businesses or corporations, her client roster is a who's who of blue-chip companies, thought leaders, CEO's, experts and inventors.

After years of launching her client's books, Erin is penning one of her own entitled: *Chasing Pretty: The Day the Fat Lady Stopped Singing,* which has an anticipated pub date in 2024.

For more information on Erin, visit:

www.theErinNetwork.com

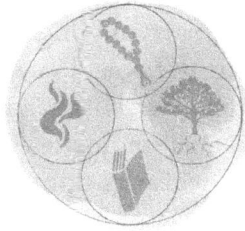

PRODUCING MINDSET

Jenna Edwards

"How selfish of you." The words rang in my head like foghorns ringing through the mist of the sea. I couldn't hold in the tears as they flowed from my eyes, leaving stains in their wake. *How could he say that?* I thought to myself. *Wasn't my response appropriate?* I mean, he said, "Nice work on the film," and my response was "Yeah, everyone did a great job." I don't understand how that's selfish. I just sat there unable to stop the tears from flowing, feeling even more insecure and, frankly, more embarrassed than I could have ever imagined.

Though I had never met this man, I know my friend had been speaking to him about my situation for months now. A horribly frustrating situation where I was thrust into a leadership position I wasn't ready for. A situation that brought up issues of abandonment and insecurity from my childhood.

You see, I grew up in conflicting environments. On the one hand, the women in my family were strong-willed and independent. Especially my mom. She was the lead singer in my parents' rock band and did all their bookings as well. To say she could carry her own would be an understatement. And, on the other hand, the town I grew up in was extremely . . . let's say, *traditional.* I felt the pressure to grow up, marry my high-school sweetheart, and have babies, regularly. But, at home, I saw the way I really wanted to be. A woman who could take charge and lead with the best of them. The issue was that my mom's take-charge attitude led to two divorces and lots of whispers from the large gossip mill in town about how selfish she was. These whispers contributed to my biggest fear: being selfish.

I definitely knew I didn't belong in that small town, so when I was old enough, I left to pursue my dream of living in Los Angeles where I dove into the film and television industry. An industry traditionally dominated by men.

Being away from my mom definitely had an effect on my self-esteem. Not having that energy of strength, courage, and, if I'm being honest, rebellion around me on a regular basis led me to a complete lack of trust in myself. And instead of being confident, I became a doormat.

Being a doormat when you're supposed to be the leader of an entire feature film is not the most effective. So, when I finally got to meet this man, a man I respected so much based on all the things I had heard about him, I was so happy. That is, until he said those words.

A little context. Two years prior, I had agreed to produce a pretty intense feature film, my first feature film as a producer. And it was no small feat. It had a really heavy subject matter, with hundreds of crew and cast members, we were filming in a strange city, and there was an incredible amount of friction between the other producer and key members of the crew. This producer had produced before, so when I signed on, I believed they would be the lead on the project and I would have an opportunity to learn the ropes from them. But, once all the friction started, the idea of learning while doing wasn't an option anymore and I was thrown into the leadership role, a role I was nowhere close to prepared to take on.

While producing this film, my doormat personality coupled

with this high-pressure environment led to more anxiety and panic than I knew what to do with. So, my nightly ritual became to literally cry myself to sleep. My friend was part of the crew, thank goodness, and witnessed these meltdowns on a daily basis and would talk with this man, her father, about it regularly. She'd then come back to me with pieces of wisdom from her phone calls, and this kept me going.

The man was deep into the self-development space and had been for years. He was super wise and, like I said, I trusted him. I trusted him enough that I pulled myself together, lifted my head, and looked him in the eye When he saw how utterly confused I was, he went on to explain what he meant.

He went on to explain that when we're in a leadership position, it's important for us to take credit for the good work we've done. If we don't, how will those who are looking to us to lead know when they are doing a good job? In addition, how will they know what healthy confidence looks like? Because confidence isn't the same as cockiness. Confident people trust the work they do and take and give credit without their ego getting in the way.

This concept blew my mind. In that moment, my entire perspective changed. I started to grasp what true leadership is. I began to understand the difference between being selfish and being a doormat, being confident and being cocky.

I decided that I would dive deep into leadership concepts, and I spent the next decade consuming everything I could on the topic. I began teaching production at a college level, and with each student experience, I leaned into, what I believe is, the key ingredient to being a great producer: focusing on what's best for the project.

Since this moment happened, I've gone on to produce and consult on over 125 film and media projects, work with some of the biggest brands and studios in the world, and give workshops and talks to thousands of people about what I think is the key mindset when collaborating—the mindset of what's best for the project?

Listen, we all have egos. My therapist likes to point out that the goal is to have a healthy ego. Let's acknowledge that idea but put it aside for the time being because the ego I'm talking about in this story is the one that gets in the way of success. And by *success,* I mean success for everyone involved. When you are collaborating with others, working as a team, and have agreed on a goal, sometimes that goal gets completely derailed because of egos. In the film industry, it's often called "creative differences."

But, if you can all come together and agree on the type of goal you're setting (or the type of project you want to produce together), it allows for everyone to remove their egos. Agreeing on and knowing exactly what you are working toward allows you to focus on and make decisions based on what's best for the project. That way, you can remove emotions and let logic take the reins. You can choose the best course of action, and it doesn't matter who had the idea.

Since adopting this mindset, it has gotten me out of more potentially sticky situations than I can count. I mean, we're all human, so logic might take a minute to prevail, but if you can ensure before you start the project that everyone on your team is aligned and committed to this one practice—the practice of focusing on what's best for the project—you will have a much more enjoyable time creating whatever it is you want to create.

I do want to point out something important from the last section, and that's the part about everyone agreeing before you start the project. I've had to come in and consult on more projects than I can count where the leaders were not on the same page. The common denominator I've noticed in all of these situations is that they didn't have the tough conversation about what each of them wanted the project to be before agreeing to work on it.

This often happens because we're afraid. Afraid that if we say the wrong thing or don't have the same idea, that we won't get brought on—essentially, we won't get the job. This brings me back to the beginning. I definitely got myself into that horrible situation because I was too afraid and insecure to have the conversation about what I wanted out of the project, and it became very clear a little too late that the other producer and our leads weren't clear about what they wanted either, and because of that, the project did not turn out the best way possible.

Because I am so acutely aware of how that fear feels and the consequences that come from it, my focus in my consulting business is on facilitating conversations, meetings, and workshops, knowing there's most likely someone in the room too afraid to speak up and it's my job to make sure they do in the most comfortable, productive way possible.

Since I love a good checklist, let me lay out my process in the hopes that you can take it and work it into your life and projects:

When I begin a group project, I will sit down with everyone beforehand and ask them what they think the goal is and what the best approach to achieving the goal is. I get a feel for how each person works and thinks. At this time, I can clarify and adjust if the person doesn't understand the goal completely.

Once we're all gathered, the first thing I do is make sure everyone is on the same page regarding the goal. I also make sure they all know that in this process, we have to remove all egos. This allows for everyone to relax a bit because we won't be caring who is making the suggestions on the course of action; instead, we will be focusing only on the suggestion itself.

In order to facilitate the discussions, I have an entire toolbox of exercises to get everyone focused on the best possible set of actions to achieve the goal. Some of the exercises are anonymous, and some are discussion based. It all depends on the group, and I base these exercises on the info I gather in the initial one-on-one conversations.

Once action steps are decided, they are written down and

handed out to everyone so that there are no question marks among the group.

My goal in my consulting business is to ensure everyone has a voice and that everyone working toward the goal is heard and contributing to how the goal can be achieved. I've been lucky in my life to work with some incredible companies, and the biggest and best of them have the same idea: that diversity in ideas, thoughts, personalities, people as a whole, are their biggest strengths. And, focusing on what's best for the project combined with highlighting everyone's strengths in how to get there is the ultimate key to success.

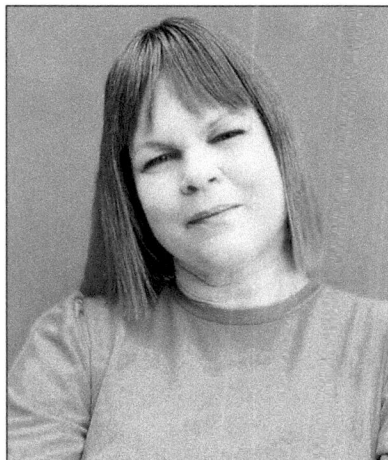

ABOUT JENNA EDWARDS

Jenna Edwards is a #1 best-selling author who has spent the past 2 decades in front of and behind the camera as an actress (*Buffy the Vampire Slayer, Malcolm in the Middle*) and producer (*April Showers*—#1 on *iTunes, In the Darkness*—the 1st narrative feature for *Hulu.com*).

Nearly being killed in the 2003 Farmer's Market crash in Santa Monica, CA led Jenna on a path to understanding mindset in order to heal her severe Post Traumatic Stress Disorder (PTSD).

Coupling this mindset work with Jenna's collaborative background, she has made her way into the exciting field of professional facilitation where she helps companies and youth leadership organizations understand not only what their goals are, but how they can work as teams to achieve them.

She is passionate about helping people uncover the best *way* to achieve their goals creating win-win experiences wherever she goes.

You can learn more about Jenna at:

www.JennaEdwards.com

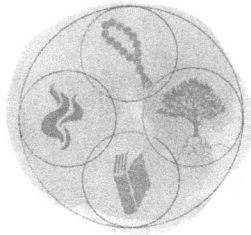

FORGET FEAR

Marisa Griffin

I n life, the most beautiful adventures and meaningful accomplishments lie just beyond the veil of fear, of self-doubt, of ourselves. It's that voice within us that either pushes us forward with determination or paralyzes us, holding us back from new experiences and personal growth. Fear of change or fear of the unknown often stops us from pursuing our dreams. But what if we chose to move forward anyway? What if we rewrote the narrative and turned that negative self-talk into courage?

We all want to live our best life, right? But, my gosh, do we get in our own way. Fear has had its firm grip on me for so long. It still plagues me and stops me in my tracks. In fact, just the other day I was crying in the car with my friend about how I wasn't sure I could do it—do the things I'm hoping to accomplish—but it was fear . . . fear holding me back, fear telling me that I'm not good enough that people might laugh at me, that my dream is silly.

So as I sit here and tell you that we need to overcome fear to move forward, trust me when I say that I'm there with you. Change and growth are fluid; they have high moments of excitement and low moments of self-doubt. I've lost count of how many times I wanted to quit. But I want to share with you what happens when you keep going, when you choose yourself, when you stop letting fear get in the way of your dreams.

So who am I? Why am I even talking about this? I'm getting there, promise, but first you have to understand who I am and why this matters so much to me.

I'm a girl living in the Midwest, married for over twenty years to my high school sweetheart, with our two kids and our two dogs in our house in the suburbs. I worked in the corporate world for a long time, took some time off to have my second baby, then went back to work. My kids are now fourteen and twenty, and as I watch them grow into adulthood and who they are meant to be, I sit here and wonder, *Am I who I am meant to be?*

I have always loved working. I've always been good at it, climbed the ladders, accepted the awards, all the things. But as with everyone else, when the pandemic hit, everything shifted. As I watched the world stop, my priorities changed. I no longer cared if I was the star employee, I no longer needed the professional accolades—what I craved more than anything was time. Time with family while we are all still together under one roof. Time with my husband as we navigate life together and watch our children grow. Time with myself to really know who I am and what I want.

I am extremely fortunate in that I have a great job with a great work family. I have work-life balance, and I work with an amazing team. However, it's not going to last forever, and it's not what I want to do forever. My boss is getting close to retirement, and there is an estimated end date to my current career. This has forced me to look forward now versus later and really think about what I want in life, what I want to pour my time and energy into. I realized what I do and don't want.

I don't want to be tied to a phone or a computer all day every day.

I don't want to do work for someone else anymore.

I want to spend my time on something I've created.

I want my days to be filled with something I'm passionate about.

I want what we all want: calendar and financial freedom.

But why does this have to be some arbitrary dream? Why can't I make this my reality? What does that even look like? I invite you to join me on this personal journey of working through fear and how it has opened the doors to countless opportunities that were more than what I had even imagined for myself.

Honestly, I started before I really knew I had. As most of us post-pandemic, I really missed people. I started to play in the online space, and while it was a way to connect with my girl-friends, it grew. I found that I really enjoyed creating those con-nections, and I really enjoyed creating content; what started as a fun online beauty group for my girlfriends turned into a small beauty business, and as that grew, I started to add more of what I enjoyed into the online space.

As it grew, my ideas grew, and I kept thinking, *Wouldn't it be nice if I could do this full-time? Wouldn't it be great if this was my actual job? Wouldn't it be fun if I could turn my hobbies into streams of income?* But it never went away—it never stopped. I was drawn to it. I could see it. I could see my future, but I had no clue how to get there.

I was so excited to get started, I went for it all: I created a blog, I set up an email subscription, I put more and more effort into my beauty business, I created a website to sell custom gift boxes and care packages, I started to post reviews on my outfits online, I started to share beauty tips and style inspiration. I just kept going and going, and slowly it started growing. I was having so much fun with it—until I wasn't.

I would research other creators and end up over consum-ing and then comparing myself to others who had been doing this much longer than I had. These creators had hundreds of thousands of followers. Their content quality was much higher than mine; clearly they had the state-of-the-art equipment that I couldn't justify purchasing. They were half my age, thinner, prettier, more vibrant, more relevant—they knew what they were doing! Who was I to try and take up space in this online world? A mom in her 40s in the Midwest? Why would anyone even care?

Fear set in, and I just wanted to quit, delete everything, and pretend it never happened. Then guess what happened. My content started to get more attention, I gained more followers, but what really mattered is people were starting to engage with my content! I was having fun again! I gave it my all and just kept going. Then fear would set in again, I would think of a million reasons to stop. Then I had a couple boutiques reach out to me; they wanted to work with me! Another high—back to fun and back to work! Then guess who would come right back. Yep, fear . . .

My beauty business was still small, but it was steady, and it was my happy place—interacting in my group was everything. It just filled my cup. But it kept coming back, fear . . . I ended up in burnout again and again. I was letting fear decide for me and slowly watching my dreams fade away. Fear was telling me that it was silly; fear was telling me that I'd never achieve what I so badly wanted. I could see it—clear as day—I could see my dream, but I just couldn't reach it.

Fear is natural. In fact, having a little fear is healthy. After all, it's about self-preservation. However, it seeps into our thoughts and creates a web of doubts, insecurities, and limiting beliefs. Fear is loud. Fear is cruel. Fear is persistent. Fear had long been my constant companion, holding me back from venturing into uncharted territory and new possibilities.

By recognizing fear as the negative voice in our heads, we can stop it in its tracks. It helps to know what specific fears are holding us back. Is it fear of failure, rejection, judgment, ridicule, criticism, change? Friend, it's those exact fears that paralyzed my dreams, leaving me trapped within the confines of my comfort zone. By acknowledging these fears, we can confront them with clarity and intention. I realized that if I wanted to truly live the life I wanted, I had to break free from these self-imposed limitations and face my fears head-on.

Fear often lies to us; it shows us a perception of reality that amplifies negative outcomes. But what if we reframed this as untapped potential or personal growth?! We can transform our fears into a source of motivation. Confronting fear requires understanding its roots. I had to dig deep within myself, examining the specific fears that held me captive. I had to be honest with myself and name them one by one, acknowledging their presence in my life, and really just sit in not only the possibility but the reality of my worst fears coming true.

Fear of failure: I didn't get it right. I made mistakes. I wasted my time. But honestly who doesn't make mistakes? Doesn't that build character? Doesn't getting it wrong teach us what we really want and don't want? Also, who said that failure is wasted time? If anything, that is valuable time well spent learning incredibly valuable lessons.

Remember that website I told you about for custom care packages and gift boxes? Yeah, that failed. I had people ask me to make them a few boxes and then created a website and stocked up on inventory before really knowing what I was doing.

Now, am I sorry I did it? Not one bit! I'm SO glad that failed! It taught me that it's more of a hobby to me, not a passion. If I had turned that into my main business and relied on that, I would have been miserable. As it is now, it's so fun, and I love when people ask me to create gift boxes for them. And that's where that belongs: in the fun part of my life.

Fear of rejection: I wasn't chosen, they didn't want me, I wasn't good enough. Okay, well, first of all, we can't all be chosen all the time, can we? Maybe it's not our moment, maybe we're not ready. Maybe there is a valid reason I wasn't chosen. Maybe if I'm chosen now, then I won't be available for what I'm really meant to do, and honestly, not being good enough is okay. There will always be someone out there who does what you want to do better, but guess what—that's their journey, and maybe it just looks better from the outside—maybe if you really took a closer look, you would do things differently. Maybe it's not better, it's just different. I realized I'd much rather be me, the real me, than some version of me made up for someone else that I can't keep up with.

Fear of judgment: People are going to judge what they don't understand. Most judgments come from people not knowing the whole story, and no one is ever going to know the entirety of our story. It is just that: OUR story. There will be people who don't understand, and that's okay. How many things are out in the world that we don't understand? The world keeps spinning and we all live our lives just the same. It is okay for them not to get it; it's not their journey. It's not meant for them.

Fear of ridicule: I like to think that as a whole, people are good. But sadly there will always be those who make life harder for others, putting people down for what they do, what they enjoy, who they are. A lot of times it has nothing to do with the person being ridiculed and everything to do with the other person and their insecurities. This is a hard one to let go of, but that's what we have to do: let it go. We take it so personally, but remember, it really isn't about us . . .

Also, keep in mind, we are not for everyone and that's okay! Never put yourself in a box for anyone else. Give yourself permission to take up space. Be yourself and not only will your people find you, but they will cheer you on every single step of the way!

Fear of criticism: As we move forward, we are going to do things wrong, we are going to make mistakes, we just don't know what we don't know. How do we learn if no one stops to tell us or show us a better way? The right people empower and encourage you as you grow. Surround yourself with those who nurture you along the way, not those who are self-serving trying to dim your light.

I was fortunate enough to get to speak to a lovely and successful creator briefly, and she shared with me how it took YEARS to get where she is and she has so much help! She might be the only person in front of the camera, but she has a whole team behind her who makes her look good! I needed that reminder: it takes time. I needed to stop comparing myself. Period.

Fear of change: Change is scary, and people aren't always good with change. What we know is familiar, and familiar is comfortable. But let's think back to where we started in life and to where we are now: how many changes have we gone through? Can you imagine life with no change? No, not all change is fun, but change is necessary. Changing is living.

By simply shifting our perspective, we lose fear and gain excitement for new possibilities; we no longer see barriers, now we see new opportunities.

Remember I said overcoming fear and going after what you want takes work? It takes a lot of work. You have to understand that real change takes time. It's not passive—it doesn't just happen—you have to take intentional action. Help yourself by creating a plan. While you may have your sights set on the end game, you need smaller, achievable goals to get you there. You'll need to take consistent action to get yourself where you want to go. No one decides they have a goal and just wakes up the next day and has achieved it. It takes time and learning. Take classes, do your research, join peer groups, learn from others, get started, and learn as you go making mistakes along the way. The best way to learn and move forward is from experience.

You know what else matters? Taking time to celebrate your progress and to live in the moment. You need to acknowledge your wins along the way and appreciate how far you have come. You started this journey, you got where you are. Do not—I repeat, do not—lower the value of what you have done because not only are you taking away from the achievement itself but you are making yourself small. Take up space, you deserve to be there. Show not just the world why, show yourself why!

Every single step big or small is what moves you forward. For those moments will teach us so much, they might even change our path to something bigger and brighter, something completely unexpected! Sometimes when you are in the thick of it, it's hard to see how far you have come. As I was preparing for this chapter and as I was challenged to put a pen to paper and write down accomplishments and milestones that I have reached since starting my journey, I saw that list and then thought about how much time, effort, thought, and pieces of me went into each one. I was stunned. I had been so hard on myself thinking I had so far to go (which I do), but oh my gosh, look how far I have come!

Please remember that the most remarkable chapters in our lives are written when we refuse to let fear hold the pen. So f*ck fear and summon your courage. Some of our biggest and brightest dreams await us in adventures we haven't even thought of yet! This is just the start.

Let your story unfold, write your chapters with bravery, and savor the remarkable journey that lies ahead. Your dreams are waiting—go and challenge yourself to try new things. You will be amazed at what you find and who you find in yourself.

Embrace the unknown, get uncomfortable. The opportunities that await you are boundless once you get out of your own way!

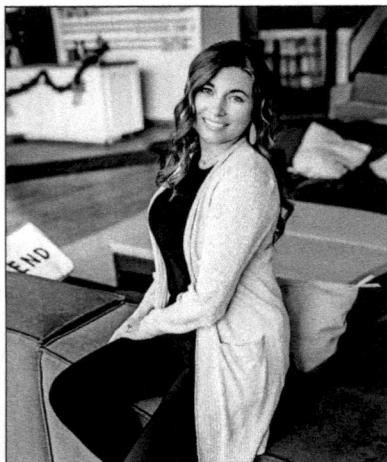

ABOUT MARISA GRIFFIN

Marisa is a multi-passionate entrepreneur, influencer, and certified online business expert. She started her business with a need and desire to connect with others and found a love for helping women feel better about themselves while showing them simple beauty and style tips, and in turn, she developed a passion for helping others find courage and confidence in themselves.

Marisa lives in Kansas City, MO, with her husband, children, and dogs. She loves to read, travel, and connect with the people in her life. To Marisa, her family and friends are everything. While she shares her love for all things beauty, style, and shopping, what matters to her the most is the adventures and life experiences that you won't find in a store.

To Connect with Marisa:

https://linktr.ee/mxmvip

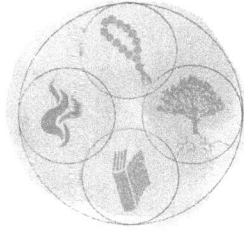

LAST PLACE NEVER FELT SO GOOD!

Erica Rasmussen

December 31, 2022—Panama Beach, Florida: I never imagined running into a new year! But, approaching 100 pounds down from my highest weight, I was on a mission to finish a running race in all fifty states. Florida was state three to check off the list. Knowing healthy habits take time to evolve into a lifestyle, I chose this goal to take better ownership of my health.

My six-year-old son begged to join me that day for the 5K race. He loved the first 0.1 miles of the 3.1-mile race, and then it got tougher. Ironically, my first running memory was as a six-year-old. I was the slowest kid on my soccer team. Even though my coach kindly let me start before everyone, I always finished last. Inward, my confidence began diminishing, with negative self-talk starting way too early in life! Outward, my B+ blood type helped fuel my enthusiasm and positivity and kindness to everyone else. It was such a dichotomy.

I struggled to fit in. By fifth grade, I refused to eat. Depression and anxiety set in. As if middle school isn't tough enough, I lost all my friends. I lost myself. I headed into my teens feeling very alone. I judged myself by my emotions. I ate lots of ice cream after school while watching TV to escape the reality of feeling insignificant, ugly, and larger than my peers. Inside I crumbled. Outside I tried staying strong.

By high school, I found outlets that gave me strength. I was one of three freshmen to make the varsity softball team. But every time I got up to bat, my confidence battle with myself took over. I got made fun of for my socks not staying up on my calves. I felt awkward. I felt alone. I got bullied. That's when bulimia set in. I hid in the art room drinking Diet Coke at lunch, painting or creating something that brought me joy in those dark high school years. I taught skiing on weekends, bringing positivity, confidence, and empowerment to so many. I still felt empty inside.

By junior year of high school, I convinced my parents to let me graduate early. My family loved me way more than I loved myself. I just wish I could've seen what I truly had to offer the world then. But I didn't. Thank God they believed in me!

Even as I began to start taking care of myself to finish high school early and lock in a spot on my college softball team, my inner light wavered. I felt so unsure of why I was even on this planet. Off I went to college in northern Vermont with my mini fridge, a laundry basket full of food, clothes, bedding, laptop, and a softball glove. I felt like a deer in headlights. But it just felt right. I had a lot of hope for a new chapter and fresh start!

My very first college class talked about types of leadership. That's when I realized I had been a leader all my life. I was a leader! Marching to the beat of my own drum was not a bad thing. So, I marched right into softball tryouts with a little more confidence. I earned a spot on the team! I was playing college softball at the age of seventeen before I even walked in my high school graduation. I felt empowered, and that felt good!

I began forming genuine friendships of a lifetime, traveling to new places, and learning what discipline for my mind and body truly meant! I was accepted for who I was, not who I wasn't. However, in my dorm room, I still struggled with food. I even moved into a room alone without a roommate; it helped me hide my eating habits. I hid it well my first semester. But by the time fall rolled around, I was diagnosed as bulimic at age eighteen. I couldn't keep it a secret anymore. My mental and physical health declined to the point of being rushed to the emergency room. That's when I had to get the help I needed. I felt like my new life was a series of waiting rooms and appointments: doctor, nutritionist, and lots of therapists. That was all a Band-Aid solution for self-love, self-confidence, and self-care.

My perseverance helped me get better. Slowly. It wasn't always easy or perfect, and I had a steep learning curve. By sophomore year, my athletic talent, positivity, and leadership earned me captain on my college volleyball team. But our very first game of the season, I collapsed on the court and was rushed away to the hospital in an ambulance. That was an expensive result of improper nutrition. (Sorry, Mom and Dad!) Truth be told, the hospital never really helped the long-term need for my mind and body to work together. It just defused the situation.

Long story short, I let my ups fuel me immensely. I gave permission for my downs to spiral my thoughts and emotions to an unhealthy place. Outward: my grit and determination shined through. Inward: I lacked true self-love. But life had to go on, so I ate through emotions, stopped regularly exercising, and gained a lot of weight. I was glad I wasn't bulimic, but I knew I had to take better care of my health.

Fast-forward a decade to when I was pregnant with my daughter: I weighed a bit shy of 300 pounds. One day, I saw obesity in my paperwork, and that ignited a fire. If I could change it, I wanted to. Not for me but for my family. They needed me!

Becoming a mom motivated me to be a better version of myself. I needed to show up for my two young kids, born about eighteen months apart. I wanted to inspire them, love them with all my heart, and show them they can be unstoppable with their goals and dreams. That meant being unstoppable with my own self-love. That meant taking better care of my mind and body.

That meant never, ever going to the hospital for a health concern I had control over. That meant I needed to continually empower myself to overcome all that dragged me down. My kids were the ultimate fuel for overcoming what had previously dragged me down. Overcoming was fuel to my fire within.

So, I worked hard, began eating smarter, and eventually became a runner. It wasn't a hobby I ever imagined enjoying. But what the mileage did for my physical and mental health fueled my zest for life again, helped me believe in myself more, and was literally what I needed to truly take ownership of my mind and body. The road still got bumpy at times, but over time I learned how much pressure I could put on myself to adequately continue on a positive path.

I had incredible mentors. I listened to their advice. I applied it. I struggled. I overcame.

Dr. Dave Braun, my most impactful mentor, told me, "Erica, you don't need rocket launchers, but you do need a parachute!" In that moment, it solved years and years of wondering why I was different, was more powerful than dozens of therapy sessions, and empowered me to think big for my future as a mom, a wife, a runner, and somebody with the ability to not only empower myself and my children but inspire others to see what's possible within them.

I knew I needed a goal that would help me sustain this ability to ignite my rocket boosters and chase my dreams while also practicing implementation of my newfound parachute. I set my sights on training for a half marathon, all while thinking it would be fun to not just start, but finish, running races in all fifty states.

That's what led me and my son to Panama Beach, Florida, on New Year's Eve of 2022. The race was extra special because Tommy joined me. He just turned six and wanted nothing more than to join me in a running race. He saw the joy I got from running. And he heard he would get a medal for finishing, which totally sealed the deal!

Already in Florida visiting family for the holidays, Tommy's "official training" began on his sixth birthday, a few days before the race. We ran on the beach at sunrise. He was so into it. He felt strong, excited, and motivated. Something about me being the slowest six-year-old on my soccer team fueled an immense desire for me to help him not feel like I did at that age. Whatever I was doing was working. He was happy and confident.

Race day came: We took our spot at the start line. I could see the glow of determination and excitement in Tommy's eyes as the race began. We ran around a small pond. "Are we done, Mom?" his cute little voice said with enthusiasm and hope. "No, honey, we just started. We have about three miles to go."

Learning from my own parents, one thing I never want as a parent is to force my kids to do something they don't want to. So, we began to walk. The race was an "out and back," which meant we got to see the racers run back by us to approach the finish. As he held back tears, Tommy said with a disappointed look, "Are we going to be last?" I told him we might be, but the best part of last place is that you get to cheer every single person on in the race. He smiled, and we began having so much fun cheering on others. It brought him so much joy as he cheered on others.

The sky got dark. It began raining. I started carrying Tommy out of pure Mom love whenever he wanted me to. Race organizers began picking up the signs behind us, and then in front of us. A golf cart with volunteers hovered behind us until eventually heading back to the start. "Next time we run a 5K, can it be a shorter one?" he asked. I smiled, and the sun came back out to bring us more hope.

In fear of the finish line being taken down before we reached it, I began jogging with Tommy on my shoulders. I wanted him to feel the accomplishment of crossing the finish line. My knees and back began to hurt, but every minute was worth it! We rounded the corner toward the finish line, and it was still there! My smile grew. After positively encouraging my son for ninety minutes, the end was in sight! Race organizers waited for us. We crossed it together, with Tommy smiling on my shoulders. Earning last place never felt so good.

That moment helped me realize everything I went through in my childhood led me to show up better for my son. It made my struggles all worth it. For him. For both my kids' futures. His mindset as a six-year-old is far different from mine at that age. I know that will strengthen his path forward. He has his own rocket boosters, and I will always be his parachute!

The truth is, we all can run toward our goals. Sometimes it's a walk, a jog, a hop, or a crawl—but we just have to move forward. One foot in front of the other. One day at a time. Sometimes one minute at a time. If we take ownership of our path forward, overcoming what holds us back becomes much easier. When we believe in ourselves, what seems impossible can become possible.

A year ago, running a mile was hard. Now, I'm training for the 26.2-mile New York City Marathon. If I get last place, it'll still be a victory. Tommy would agree.

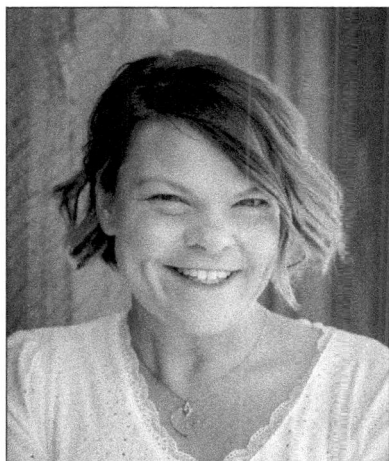

ABOUT ERICA RASMUSSEN

Erica Rasmussen is a goal-getter from Gunnison, Colorado. A speaker, coach, mom, wife, and true believer in the power of positivity, Erica is on a mission to complete a running race in all fifty states. Down roughly 100 pounds from her highest weight, Erica has taken ownership of her mind and body to truly run for her goals.

Learn more about Erica and her journey at:

RunForYourGoals.com

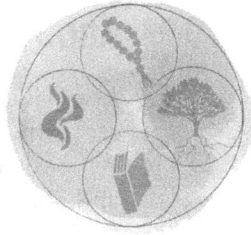

LOST AND FOUND

Tiffany Donovan Green

With his muscular hand at the back of my neck, he guided me forward. I was both eager and anxious as we inched our way toward the entrance. A small line had formed, and we could hear the shrieks of the brave souls ahead of us. I was just a few months shy of my thirteenth birthday. My father, with whom I was obligated to spend the afternoon, had offered to treat me to an activity of my choosing. He was always looking for ways to assuage the guilt he felt after the divorce.

It was mid-October, and Halloween festivities were in full swing. At a shopping mall in suburban Detroit on a sunny Saturday afternoon, I stood with my dad before a make-shift house of horrors. An innocent preteen giddy with excitement and anticipation, I was oblivious to the event that was about to unfold and haunt my journey into adulthood.

We entered through a black fabric curtain with a small group of fellow spectators, a mix of adults with small children, young couples, and a few rowdy older teens. Moving cautiously in the darkness through a smoky graveyard, we squealed in unison when various monsters lurched from the shadows. A vignette featuring a butcher's shop of human remains was particularly gruesome and caused me to question my insistence on this particular activity. I could sense my father's anxiety; he pulled me closer, his grip on the back of my neck tightened. We fell to the end of the procession.

The combination of dry ice and utter darkness was claustrophobic. As we progressed through the amusements, I was eager for the next ghoulish attraction so that my sight would return. My dad directed me from behind, his hands now steering my shoulders as his feet continuously clipped the back of my heels. We shuffled forward, step after step, through the unlit maze, and although I felt comforted by his presence and authority, an uneasiness accumulated in the pit of my stomach. Forging through the thick lightlessness, I slowly became cognizant that we were alone, separated from the group. We were lost. For twenty minutes or more, we wandered between curtains and rods, relying on distant screams and the sense of touch to guide us in the absence of vision.

At one point, a man's face appeared in the abyss, illuminated by a dim flashlight; it seemed to float in thin air as he motioned us to follow him. For some odd reason, my father declined and pushed me onward. "Daddy, that's our guide. Follow him!" I pleaded, but it was too late. Darkness descended as the guide dropped the curtain, leaving us in total blindness.

We all have moments that matter, moments that influence our trajectory, that guide the evolution of our character, and even cement our fate. Sometimes, the perception of these moments is instantaneous, identifiable within a heartbeat, and engraved forever in our senses.

Other times, these moments are perceived only in hindsight, after deliberate reflection and the kind of understanding that develops with life experience. They take shape incrementally, coming into focus as our awareness grows, like fluid lines on a blank canvas that gradually become recognizable under the pen of a skilled artist.

For me, the metaphorical significance of the haunted house was delayed. Initially, when I first emerged from the tangle of pipe and drape that formed the backstage of the amusement, I was simply annoyed that I missed half the show because I was steered in the wrong direction and failed to seize the opportunity to correct course; but over time, I found cause to reexamine the experience and identify it as an important turning point in my life.

In retrospect, I recognize that the incident also gained import because it coincided with the drama associated with becoming a young adult. Puberty—that radical hormone infusion that forces a transformation of both body and mind—is akin to rebirth. The individuality and confidence of the self-assured child gives way to teenage self-doubt and the need for peer acceptance; the pressure to conform coupled with a rebellious testing of limits and exploration of new terrain results in a metamorphosis that disconnects the individual from prepubescent identity prior to full adult self-actualization. It was in this emotionally tumultuous no man's land of teen angst that I found myself stranded in that lightless void, at a crossroads between childhood and maturity, blindly stepping foot toward a new frontier.

I'd like to think that we have the power to choose the moments that matter and that we can control, shape, and carefully curate our memories to preserve the most precious and meaningful ones. By cultivating the memory of milestone events—a heart-felt celebration, a first kiss, a graduation, a college acceptance, a romance, first day on the job, a wedding, a promotion, birth of a child, a new home, baby's first steps, and so forth—we can paint a picture of a charmed life.

Unfortunately, we do not have complete control over the neural circuitry that preserves our remembrances any more than we have complete control over the varied and often unpredictable circumstances that make up daily life. It's the universality of human vulnerability that teaches us empathy and perseverance, subjecting us to struggle and defeat in the pursuit of love and happiness.

Although some may be more skilled than others when it comes to focusing on the positive, I believe we are also genetically wired to remember distressing and emotion-provoking events. Our brain absorbs this information, and in an effort to protect us, employs defenses rooted in a complex biology that result in anxiety, distrust, and other forms of emotional conditioning.

At the time, I did not think of the haunted house experience as particularly traumatizing despite the initial anxiety it provoked. But over time, I became increasingly reminiscent of the ordeal. Whenever I felt like I had hit a dead-end or I began questioning my choices, I was transported in time to that house of horrors, to what it felt like to be lost in the dark, not knowing which way to turn, stymied by doubt and indecision. I relived the sensation of airlessness derived from an awareness of being off-track, and I imagined myself stranded on an invisible path toward an unknown future. It was less a fear of the dark than it was a fear of making the wrong move, missing out, and squandering opportunity. My memory of getting stuck behind the scenes morphed into a metaphor for being stuck in real life, boxed in by my own choices, trapped by a series of decisions I supported, leading me to conclude that ultimately, I'm responsible for my own mess.

Hindsight is like the punch line of a clever joke. That "aha" moment operates like a light switch: the moment import is revealed, the tension produced by the anticipation dissipates, and irony is acknowledged by shared appreciation in the form of a hardy chuckle.

Hindsight. It's relatable. We've all been there. Now that the outcome is visible, it seems so obvious. But a joke is only successful when the punchline is unpredictable, catches us off-guard, and avoids mundane clichés. Hindsight functions in much the same way in that it depends on the unknown, and its significance is revealed only after we have succumbed to the unforeseen hazard.

When I find myself in self-doubt, contemplating my choices with the benefit of hindsight, lost in that house of horrors trying to decipher when and where I went off course, it's easy to wallow in the "if onlys" and "what ifs," to attribute blame to others, and surrender to fear and regret. But then I recall the moment when I emerged from the backstage curtain onto an avenue of glittering lights emanating from the storefronts in that indoor suburban mall, and I rediscover my power. It took me years to get there, but I eventually learned, and likely will continue to learn, the lessons of that experience, the most important of which is how to see in the dark.

As a small child, I wore a red cape and raced around the neighborhood pretending to accomplish feats of heroism, but it was my mother who was the real hero. An ardent feminist and outspoken human rights and environmental activist, she cultivated in me values underscoring empathy, dignity, and justice. This upbringing became the foundation of my confidence, resilience, and self-worth. But divorce fractured our family, and in the absence of emotional support, my mother succumbed to the stress of raising two children on her own. Her health began to fail, so I strapped on my cape and came to the rescue. I took on an inappropriate amount of responsibility at too young an age, feeling obligated to protect everyone and everything around me. The need to assert order and control to protect my mother and baby brother led to a hypervigilance to make the right choice. But how? There were infinite paths before me; I could only guess where each would lead. It was the same quandary I would later experience in the haunted house: I was alone in the dark.

Perhaps if I had not sought adventure that fateful Halloween, had I not ventured into the "Castle of Fright" with my father, and had we not become separated from the guide and forced to find footing in an off-trail environment, I may not have come to terms with my challenging childhood and may not have grown to become a pillar of strength in my own family. I realize now that the haunted house experience was simply a metaphorical representation of a childhood trauma that had already taken place. I had been there before. In fact, I was lost before I even arrived.

I'm sold on that timeless adage that can be roughly restated:

You must be lost before you can be found. Throughout the course of our lives, we are in the making, molded by circumstance and our ability to comprehend our significance and purpose. In the depths of that house of horrors, after the disappearance of the tour guide, after I lost confidence in my father, and when my anxiety was at its apex, followed a moment of acceptance and peace. In that instance, I became aware not only of my singularity but of a higher power, a universal intelligence that obligated me to silence my mind and consult my other senses. Reassured by an awakened sense of self, I calmly took the lead. I was no longer driven externally, rather I forged a path through my own volition and internal wisdom. I think of it as my Jedi moment. By releasing control, I gained it. I let go, shifted my focus, and discovered a force inside me, an innate sensibility that revealed the way. I found a light in the darkness.

When I look back on the sense of empowerment that derived from this experience, I feel obliged to share my discovery with those who find themselves at a crossroads. Hidden deep inside our bones is a readily accessible intelligence with ancient origins rooted in love, patience, and understanding. To access it, it is necessary to silence the mind, accept the present moment, and allow the internal compass to lead. Although I am still prone to questioning my choices, hoping that my decisions are fruitful, trusting my instincts and acknowledging that there is more than one path toward purpose relieves my anxiety and self-doubt. When I find myself in circumstances that tempt me towards despair, I remember the haunted house and the superpower that lives inside me—that lives inside each of us like an internal flashlight. By following our own navigation system, we have the ability to change course at any moment and create a new reality with fresh opportunities. Education and experimentation will help to circumvent roadblocks and aid reinvention. Seek guidance, if necessary, but avoid being steered by others. This is your journey. You have the power to correct course. The possibilities are infinite.

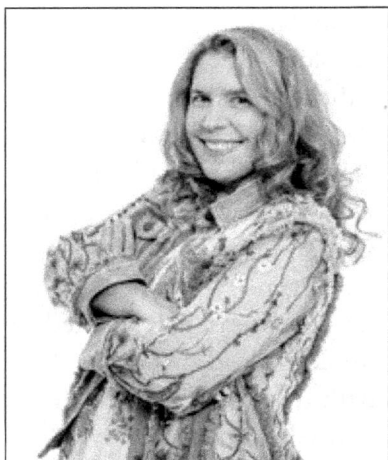

MEET TIFFANY DONOVAN GREEN

Tiffany Donovan Green is an educated professional lawyer, interior designer, event organizer and an entrepreneur, whose creative well runs very deep. An energetic and multifaceted person, she is driven by a need to find outlets for her many interests and her passion for artistic expression.

The enterprises Tiffany has founded include The Green House Interiors, specializing in healthy sustainable design; The Global Preservation Society, a 501(c)(3) organization dedicated to environmental stewardship and sustainability; and The Tiara Club, a 501(c)(3) organization dedicated to women's self-empowerment.

Tiffany earned a Bachelor of Arts in History and Political Science from Albion College in Albion, MI, a Master of Arts in History at Oakland University in Rochester, MI, and a Juris Doctorate/LLM in International and Comparative Law from Cornell Law School in Ithaca, NY. She is currently finishing a Master of Arts in Interior Design and Architecture at Fairfield University in Fairfield, CT. She has also taken on the role of author for a book in the series published by Kate Buter, *Women Who Dream*, and *Dear Younger Self*, both of which enjoy a best-seller ranking. She lives in southwestern Connecticut with her husband and their two children.

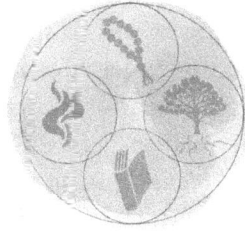

MOMENT, I CHOOSE ME

Danielle Lynn

I am ready to tell my readers it is okay to choose you!

My story is a difficult but very relatable one to share. Wanting to be a mother and have a family of my own was a dream I once had. To even say or write the words "once desired" is exceedingly difficult for me. This dream and desire fell short as I struggled with recurrent miscarriages.

Statistics say one out of four pregnancies end in miscarriage or a pregnancy loss. I personally have experienced the struggles of infertility and have had five miscarriages. I do believe I have had other early pregnancy losses but nothing that was proven with a positive pregnancy test nor ultrasound. All my miscarriage experiences have been completely different, even though the outcome was the same: I had lost my child. Dreams of your child's future and family events come to an end. Hurt, heartache, anger, and worry all set in. This entire process becomes an emotional roller-coaster, with no end in sight. Grief is so emotional and difficult to process. While I have had ongoing grief and hurt, I knew I needed the time to heal. As a counselor, I understand all too well the importance of self-care. This healing I needed was different. It was more about coming to terms with choosing myself again.

Part of my healing process was to speak, guide, and support other women who have also experienced infertility, miscarriage, and child loss. The moment I chose me was during a time of distress and emotional grief and loss. In 2019, I released the book *Silent Grief, Healing, and Hope*. During the time I was compiling and working on my publication, I experienced my fifth miscarriage. As I shared personal experiences of heartache and loss after loss with my readers and anyone close to me, I began to feel a shift in my thoughts. I began to feel a change on the inside, and I began to worry, as a woman, what having numerous miscarriages could do to my body. What about my mental health? I became so focused on trying to become a mother and working through the difficulties emotionally that I began to lose sight of who I was. I began to lose the ideas of other possibilities for my future. I began to feel a wall with my spouse emotionally. I wanted to reconnect with him. I wanted to reconnect with myself. I needed me and us back! I had come to terms with choosing myself again.

After my last pregnancy loss, I had a doctor's appointment to do a complete all over health check with my hormones, my thyroid function, and a complete breast exam, including a mammogram and ultrasound. I went to a new doctor in the women's center located in Wexford, PA. I had so many questions and concerns about how my body was handling the constant hormone changes in a short amount of time. As I went over my history of miscarriages and other family health concerns, the doctor explained something to me that caused me to worry—still concerns me to this day!

The doctor thoroughly reviewed my health and history of miscarriages, placing me at 38.6% risk of developing breast cancer. Based on family history of cancers, my risk level added another 22.4% of an increase in developing breast cancer. A women's doctor explained the health concern for females with our hormones, pregnancy loss, and the connection of our uterus and ovaries with the hormones of the female breast. In all, I am at a 61% risk of developing breast cancer! This extremely high percentage scared me! It has made me think about completing genetic testing for breast cancer and how I need to stay up to date with my annual check-ups. With my risk being so high, I am examined and monitored every six months for a mammogram and breast ultrasound. My doctors continue to encourage me to do genetic testing. This is something I have not completed, due to the worry of the test results. I do believe one day I will complete the genetic testing though so that I do not have to complete the thorough examinations every six months.

After this appointment, I have made more of an effort for my overall health and well-being. I began to refocus on how I need to take care of my body and make my needs a priority within my life. I needed to really understand what my body physically went through, especially in having D&C procedures. Most of the pregnancy losses resulted in this procedure due to my uterus not recognizing the pregnancy loss. My uterus continued to grow during two of the miscarriages. I have been concerned about the possibility of early onset menopause, a diagnosis of breast cancer, struggling with my metabolism, and inflammation issues that often lead to autoimmune disorders or a thyroid diagnosis.

The importance of seeing my primary care physician and specialist is always needed. Following through on my medical concerns was the start of putting me first again! I was not seeing a doctor about trying to become pregnant or because of a miscarriage. I was not lying in bed crying with worry of the unknown. I was making an honest effort to check into my medical health needs and concerns for *me*.

Watching my nutritional needs has also played more of a significant role, but we all know how difficult it can be eating healthy consistently. I'm learning to eat mostly protein, fruits, and veggies, and working to avoid sugar still to this day! Keeping my stress level in check is one of the things I need to always maintain. If we are under extreme distress, our cortisol levels spike, and it is difficult to maintain a healthy weight or lose weight, often causing issues with our thyroid. I have learned about the benefits of gut health these last four-plus years, and taking the right supplements for our health is extremely beneficial. Being on a good prebiotic, probiotic, and magnesium supplement continues to help strengthen and maintain my gut health, as well as my mental health. I have easily recognized how food affects my stress and level of anxiety. Studies show that 70–90% of how we feel comes from our gut! If I eat a lot of carbohydrates, I am tired and feel more sluggish. If I eat a lot of sweets, chocolate, and desserts, my acid reflux returns and my anxiety returns.

Unresolved emotional issues can also result in medical issues. As a counselor, I understand all too well what happens emotionally and physically to our mind and bodies if we suppress anything causing us emotional distress. It is important to talk to someone you trust. Finding a counselor or therapist for additional support is always helpful as well. What I have learned in the last twenty-four years of being a social worker, counselor, or therapist is that having the support of someone not within your personal life helps you look at your problems differently. Get a support network different from family, friends, and peers. A counselor or therapist will help you process your emotions, support you where you are with your problems and unresolved issues without being personally involved. Loved ones usually want to instantly help the person to feel better and will often tell them what they want to hear. Outside support helps you process and problem solve where you are without giving you answers to fix your problems.

Throughout my healing journey, I also wanted to reconnect with my husband and get us back. I could feel our relationship struggle. I could see my relationship struggling with the lack of connection with my husband. Feeling agitation, going through the difficulties of our emotions together, and arguing about any and everything within the relationship turned it from being supportive, fun, loving, and healthy to toxic. This is not why I married my husband! He was my best friend and still is today! I was feeling so unhealthy mentally, emotionally, and physically. I needed to stop focusing on the idea of having a baby, a family, and learn to re-love and give myself grace and time to heal. I needed to heal emotionally: I was afraid of attachment in each pregnancy because of the end results.

The future my husband and I were planning was no more. I decided to stop trying to have a family and learn to appreciate the life and family I have! I continue to learn to appreciate my husband and his sacrifices within our relationship.

During this moment, I learned how powerful it became to refocus on my goals, and I knew I needed to choose me again! I began revisiting many areas of my life that were always important to me and began to revisit these areas: self-care, personal growth, professional development, gratitude, relationships, and being physically strong and healthy, and I returned to writing, reconnecting, and finding the Lord! I began to make an honest effort to read the Bible and understand His Word. I found the importance of connection again with friendships and looked for online Christian support. I began to explore various opportunities, passion, and energy on personal achievements. When my life is unbalanced, I need to revisit any of these areas of my life and work on what I am avoiding: regaining balance. To be honest, I am continuing to heal and put myself first again.

Ultimately, your happiness and fulfillment are the most important factors to consider when making life choices. So, embrace your decision to prioritize yourself and your dreams, and live your life to the fullest, knowing that you have chosen the path that feels right for you. I am here to tell you that it is okay to choose you again! It is okay to stop trying to fit into societal norms of becoming a mother or having a family because you are a female. It is okay to not want to be a mother. It is okay to always put yourself first so you can make a positive impact within your family, in your place of employment or career, or for yourself! It is okay and is needed to have the tough conversation with your husband or partner if you are feeling that you need to stop trying to become pregnant. Be open about your feelings because you are being open and honest with your needs. Communicate openly about your decision and share your reasons, as this will help foster understanding and acceptance with your spouse or partner. No matter what, how you feel and what you want in life is important. We always need to take care of ourselves and be okay for life to unfold how it was meant to be.

Philippians 4:13 NIV

I can do all this through him who gives me strength.

ABOUT DANIELLE LYNN

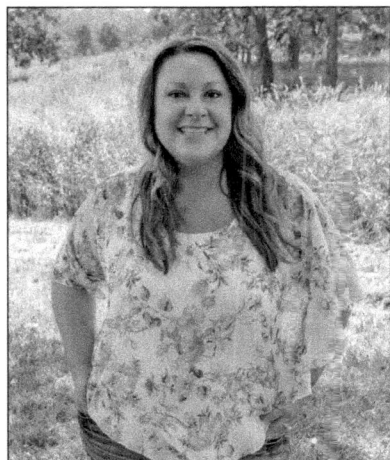

Danielle Lynn, originally from New Castle Pennsylvania, resides in East Palestine, Ohio, with her husband. Danielle earned a Bachelor of Science degree through Slippery Rock University and holds a master's degree in social work through the University of Pittsburgh. She is currently a support coach for new authors and is an addictions counselor in Pennsylvania. Danielle is also a four-time best-selling author on Amazon!

Danielle had her first solo publishing experience in 2019 with an inspirational planner, focusing on the teachings of gratitude and the use of personal photography. Also in 2019, Danielle compiled and published *Silent Grief, Healing, and Hope*. Her book became a #1 best seller in the United States and an international best seller in Germany and Canada. *Silent Grief, Healing and Hope* is fifteen inspirational stories of infertility, miscarriage, and child loss. Bringing awareness of the struggles of infertility and pregnancy loss has been very important to Danielle as she has personally experienced five miscarriages.

This has led her to help new inspiring authors to also share their story and work through their healing journey.

To connect with Danielle

www.daniellelynn.org
4daniellelynn@gmail.com
Instagram: www.Instagram.com/dschotzie

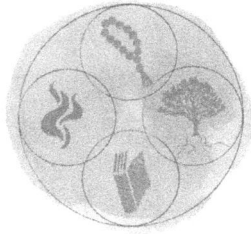

RECREATIONAL THERAPY MADE MY
LIFE WORTH LIVING

Danny W. Pettry II

Teenage years can be turbulent. This was definitely true for me.

The girl I had been dating in 1999 decided to dump me and date someone new right before her senior prom. They were engaged to be married before the end of the year. I was a year older than her, nineteen years old at this time. People often experience the stages of grief after a breakup. I felt heartache, abandonment, and despair. This experience was an existential crisis for me. I didn't know if I even wanted to live anymore. I felt uncertain about life and what direction to go. It was a rough time.

I went to a psychiatrist after the breakup. I was diagnosed with clinical depression and anxiety disorder. It made sense. I often felt down in the dumps and extremely nervous in social situations even before the breakup.

But life goes on. I was preparing to start my junior year of college in the fall of 1999. I felt like a zombie going through the motions of living. My parents wanted me to major in nursing. It was good advice. The world will always need nurses. I'd be able to make a living on nursing wages.

Forty-hours of volunteer work was required before I could be admitted to the nursing degree program at my local hometown college in Beckley, West Virginia. My cousin Tracey was a physical therapist (PT) at a rehabilitation hospital in Huntington, West Virginia, at the time. She invited me to spend a week with her to complete my forty hours of volunteer work at her hospital. Getting two hours away from my little town for a week during the summer of 1999 seemed like a good distraction.

Nurses are heroes. I shadowed them on my first day of volunteer work and discovered that they are the backbone of healthcare. However, I knew nursing wasn't right for me. It didn't make my heart sing. I felt discouraged thinking about my potential future as a nurse.

I heard people laughing in a backroom on my second day of work. This shocked me. Most of the people at this hospital were in pain. I thought the "PT" for physical therapy actually meant "painful things." How could people be having a good time here?

Naturally, I decided to go and check it out. This was the moment I discovered the wonderful world of recreational therapy.

Recreational therapists work under the supervision of an attending physician to assess and provide a mix of activity-based interventions to help people maintain and improve their social, physical, cognitive, emotional, spiritual, and overall independence and quality of life.

People are admitted to rehabilitation after an injury or disabling condition, things like strokes, traumatic brain injuries, amputations by accident or surgery. They were learning to regain skills in order to return to the highest level of functioning and independence as possible.

Wheelchair gardening was provided to allow people an opportunity to be physically active and to socialize with others. Arts and crafts were provided to help people improve fine motor skills or learn to use a non-dominant hand after a stroke or injury. Relaxation therapy was provided on the back deck under the trees with music and guided imagery. Aquatics therapy was provided in a small pool to help people build balance and coordination. Mind-challenging activities were provided to help people improve cognitive abilities.

Why were they laughing? No one could think of a country that started with the letter U. The recreational therapist ended up writing "Yugoslavia" on the dry erase board. One gentleman who had difficulty with his speech had written a message, asking the recreational therapist if he had heard of the United States of America. The group was laughing because no one (patients or staff) had thought of the USA. It was a great time. People were enjoying themselves.

I ended up spending the rest of my volunteer experience transporting people in wheelchairs to and from recreational therapy. I assisted the recreational therapists with setting up supplies or cleaning the activity room.

A Fourth of July cookout was provided to help people maintain social interaction and spend quality time with their families (and other patients). I assisted with serving food and drinks to patients during this event, carefully observing dietary needs for people who required specialized diets, like no sugar, or only soft, puréed foods.

Helping people through recreational therapy felt amazing. It is definitely intrinsically rewarding.

After that week, I knew I had to become a recreational therapist. I immediately transferred to Marshall University in Huntington, West Virginia, because they offered a degree program in therapeutic recreation. I graduated in August 2002 after completing an internship training program. I was grateful to be hired as a recreational therapist on August 12, 2002, at a psychiatric hospital for their Psychiatric Residential Treatment Facilities (PRTF) programs. I was hired one day after completing my internship (for skilled nursing and acute care psychiatry) at a local medical center. I earned my national certification to practice in recreational therapy after taking my national written exam as soon as I could after graduation.

My work for the PRTF programs over the last twenty years has primarily consisted of helping children and teens who have experienced trauma and abuse. Some of them have had other issues, including mood disorders like depression and anxiety, attention deficit hyperactivity disorder, oppositional defiant disorder, obesity, substance abuse/chemical dependency, attachment needs, Autism Spectrum Disorder, intellectual disabilities, physical aggression, family dysfunction, and other needs.

My work has had a positive impact on children, teens, and their families in the PRTF programs.

It may appear to an outsider that these children and teens are simply participating in fun, games, and activities.

Recreational therapy isn't about the activity.

Recreational therapy is about the outcomes.

Children and teens have gained a variety of skills from my work.

They learn activities they can do to cope with stress and relax; to identify their own values, strengths, and interests; to identify activities they enjoy to cheer up and regulate their emotions. They also learn assertiveness skills opposed to verbal and physical aggression and to set healthy boundaries with others, safety skills (to protect themselves from abuse) and to identify healthy adults in their support system, social skills needed to interact with others through team building activities, physical fitness activities, healthy activities they can do to cope with trauma reminders or urges to self-harm, use substances, or to distract themselves when wanting to act out aggressively.

I wanted to learn and grow as a professional. I wanted to be the best I can be in my world. I decided to earn a Master of Science degree from Indiana University (IU), which has one of the nation's leading recreational therapy degree programs. I maintained full-time work as a recreational therapist while pursuing my master's degree through IU's distance education program. I graduated in 2006.

I created Rec Therapy Today, an online continuing education program, in 2007 to help recreational therapists earn credits to renew their national certification and licenses to practice. Thousands of recreational therapists from around the world have taken courses through the program.

Recreational therapists may have a difficult time attending and participating in a national conference to earn the continuing education credits to stay relevant in the profession. One recreational therapist living on an Army base in Germany with her husband earned her credits through the program. One person was bringing recreational therapy to children in Africa. She was able to earn credits through Rec Therapy Today. Recreational therapists have described Rec Therapy Today as a "lifesaver."

These recreational therapists are able to keep their knowledge and skills relevant and refreshed so they can have a positive impact for the people who they provide services for.

These recreational therapists work in a variety of settings including psychiatric hospitals, physical rehabilitation hospitals, nursing homes, schools, the community, prisons and corrections facilities, and specialized facilities.

The recreational therapy profession has definitely made my life worth living. I probably wouldn't have discovered the profession had my girlfriend never broken up with me in 1999. I would have completed my volunteer work in nursing in Beckley and may not have discovered recreational therapy. It's cliché to say, but it was really like a beautiful lotus flower growing out of the mud.

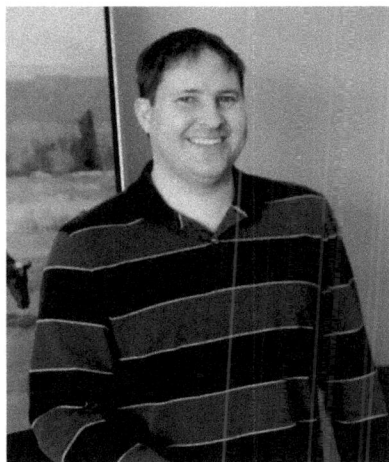

ABOUT DANNY W. PETTRY II

Danny W. Pettry II is an award-winning recreational therapist and is widely recognized as one of America's leading authorities in recreational therapy.

Danny is the creator of the Rec Therapy Today brand. He's always looked for pioneering ways to bring continuing education to recreational therapists everywhere since founding his program in 2007.

Danny has two graduate degrees, including a Master of Education in Mental Health Counseling from Lindsey Wilson College (Columbia, Kentucky) in 2012 and a Master of Science in Recreational Therapy from Indiana University (Bloomington, Indiana) in 2006. His undergraduate degree is in therapeutic recreation from Marshall University (Huntington, West Virginia) in 2002.

Danny has been a Certified Therapeutic Recreation Specialist (CTRS) since 2003. He earned Behavioral Health Specialization as an extension of his CTRS credential in 2018. He's been a National Certified Counselor (NCC) since 2013, a Licensed Professional Counselor (LPC) since 2015, and a Certified Success Principles Trainer since 2018.

Danny is a lifetime member of the American Therapeutic Recreation Association, which has awarded him with the Recreational Therapy Advocate of the Year designation in 2005 and a National Certificate of Recognition in 2018.

Connect with Danny

www.RecTherapyToday.com
Facebook: www.facebook.com/RecTherapyToday
Instagram: www.instagram.com/RecTherapyToday

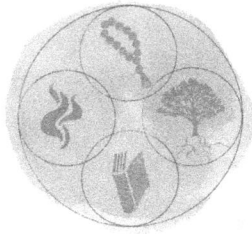

THE MOMENT

Michelle Picking

Moments—defined as a small or brief period of time. We all have them, all sorts of them. Moments of laughter, moments of sadness, insignificant ones, huge ones, ones that seem so fleeting we wonder if they really happened, while others seem to linger on. How many of you have had all of these? How many of you have had "THE MOMENT" in your life, in one regard or another? How would you describe it? Has it changed you? Would you change something in your life if you had known about it? Well, let me share my moment with you . . .

This is a love story of sorts, but it's also about realizing the choices and moments we have in our lives may not have significance at the time we make them, but ultimately, they can lead to some major events. My current husband and I have known each other for about forty years—most of our lives honestly. We grew up in the same small town and did all of the same things: went to our small festival, went to the same elementary school, we both played ball for our town, just to name a few.

When we were teenagers (fifteen and eighteen), we dated for a while. We would go to all the local festivals, I'd watch him play baseball, we'd hang out with our group of friends by the creek and go swimming. He was my first serious relationship, and I thought we'd last forever. Yeah, I know, young love. Well, it wasn't meant to be. The summer after I turned sixteen, my family moved to North Carolina. When I told him we were moving, he didn't say anything. Not a word. Not "It's okay, we'll make it work." Just nothing. My sixteen-year-old heart was SHATTERED. I didn't want to go anyway, and this was the icing on the cake. For the next two years of school (my last two years), I didn't really date. I had always been active in sports and was a cheerleader as well, but I didn't do any of that in those years. Didn't go to prom either.

Sometimes, though, there's a connection between people that neither time nor distance nor any event can break. I had moved back home for a short period of time around the time I was nineteen. During this time, I had knee surgery and wasn't supposed to be driving—especially a stick shift—but I decided to do it anyway because I needed to get out of the house for a bit. I chose to go to the bowling alley I worked at. As I was struggling to get out of the car with my crutches, I heard, "Why don't you just hand them to me, and I'll carry you in?" Now, I hadn't told anyone where I was going except my grandmother since that's where I was staying. Yet, there he was. And when I decided to head home, guess who showed up to help me get to my car and then followed me home? Yep, it was him again.

This connection has always been present between us. It can be uncanny at times, but I always felt like it was there for a reason, like something higher than we could ever see was at work. When I would come home from North Carolina to visit my family, he was always showing up unexpectedly. I would tell my family when I was coming home, but that was all, and no one ever really knew what time to expect me. I'd stop for gas, and there he would be.

I started dating someone else, and when I got married, I knew deep down it wasn't right. There were red flags—like when he left me for a past girlfriend for a month, but then came back when she left him again. When you're in a relationship, sometimes you want it to work so badly, if for no other reason than to prove yourself wrong. I won't say we didn't have good times, because we did, and for those, I'll always be grateful. He taught me a lot of skills that I still use today. But there comes a time when the bad days just outnumber the good by so much. The constant walking on eggshells because I didn't know what might set him off became such a strain on me physically and mentally. Having to always defend myself, like if I was late getting out of work or if I had to go in early, the way he would question me was like being interrogated, but yet, I wasn't allowed to ask him questions. If I did, he either shut down and wouldn't talk to me at all or the opposite would happen and it would lead to a fight where I was on the receiving end of the blows.

I remember leaving him, and when I told my family about it, I was told that I needed to go back because "he's the best thing that's ever happened to you." He was like Jekyll and Hyde: one face for the public but another in private. There were so many things that I should've paid attention to beforehand, but I chose not to. However, being in that relationship, dealing with all the pain and the abuse showed me what I DID NOT want in a relationship. It also helped to create and shape the person I am today because dealing with the level of self-loathing, non-existent self-esteem, and lack of confidence I had coming out of that relationship could have sent me down a very different path. I've learned that having a backbone and being allowed to think for myself is something that I'll never allow anyone to take away from me again.

When I remarried, there were red flags again, but once again, I chose to ignore them. Sometimes we choose to see only what we need to in any particular moment or situation. Friendship is one thing, but marriage is another completely separate dynamic for some. He was a great guy. We had been friends for years. But his thoughts of marriage and mine were drastically different. Again, we had great times. We traveled together and had so much in common. But ultimately, our goals and individual needs didn't meet where they should've in order to stay a couple. It was during this time I realized I wanted to move back home. I'd been away from home and my family for a long time, almost twenty years, and I felt the pull to get back; this was not something he was interested in doing. We separated and divorced as friends, and I'm grateful for that. It wasn't perfect, but it was the best thing to do. Again, learning more about myself and what I wanted in a partner and marriage are things I walked away with.

When I moved back home, I reached out to my now husband and told him I had moved back. He was married at the time, but we knew we'd always have our friendship and could count on each other no matter what. I had just come out of a relationship of about nine or ten months when he called and said he had left his wife because he couldn't take being in the marriage anymore and he needed to talk with someone, and I was that someone. So, I went down to see him and talk with him. We might go for a walk or have dinner or sometimes we'd just sit and talk. One night we went to our old stomping grounds at one of the local festivals we used to go to, and I was able to see and chat with his parents again.

Almost two years later, I ended up getting injured at work. What I thought was a minor accident turned into a very lengthy ordeal with five surgeries, a year and a half of physical therapy, and a ton of changes to my lifestyle. He and I weren't married at this time and hadn't even fully discussed it all, but he was by my side every step of the way. He took me to every therapy appointment, recheck at the doctor or surgeon, he was with me for my surgeries, the nerve blocks, and even when I gained weight, he never stopped being in my corner. He supported my decisions to stop the pain medications when they didn't work or made me feel worse; we talked through having the last surgery and whether it was worth it. On days when I didn't think I could handle anything else, he was by my side believing in me and telling me WE would do it together, no matter what it was or what the outcome was going to be.

About two weeks prior to my last surgery, he took me to one of our favorite places, the ball fields in our hometown where we both played as kids and where we spent a lot of time while we were dating, and he proposed.

When all of the pushback I was getting from some family about the wedding was causing me stress and I was starting to hate it all, he proposed we do it OUR way. So six months later, we got married in a very small but beautiful ceremony on a hill by the lake where we spent time growing up as well. When I say small, I mean seven people including us. But the location and the day couldn't have been any more perfect than it was on that day—a moment for us.

Let's fast-forward now to where we are currently having celebrated our eighth wedding anniversary and more than a decade of being together. During this time, we've had so many ups and downs—like most marriages—but the unconditional support that is found on both sides is unmatched. He is the one I want and I have the amazing chance to share all the things with: the good, the bad, the ugly. He's my grounding point. He's the voice on the end of the phone when I need to share tough news or a rough situation with. He's the voice who celebrates with me when the good things happen. He's the one I need a hug from when it feels like everything is going wrong or I feel overwhelmed. He's also the one who pushes me each day to become the best version of myself.

The support we share knows no boundaries. When he decided to retire from a job of thirty-three and a half years to start over doing the same thing in a different location, he asked me if I thought he was crazy. I told him, "Absolutely not, this is what you love to do and you have an amazing opportunity, so take it." He needed classes to get a certification. My words were "Go do it." This is where his passion lies and he's amazing at it, so there's not a place or a reason why I wouldn't support him in doing whatever it is he needs in order to be successful and grow in it. And the best thing is that all of that support is reciprocated 1,000-fold back to me. Whether it's my jump back into my career, my lifting and competition or running the personal training business, he believes in me and pushes me to go after whatever my dream or crazy idea may be.

When it comes to my competition schedule, he gets to choose the one(s) he would like to attend since he can't be at them all due to his vacation time and schedule. Last year, he chose to come to Puerto Rico with me. The one thing he said he wanted to do was swim in the ocean—not all the tourist stuff, just swim in the warm ocean water. Lying on the beach, watching my husband swim in the warm ocean water with a huge grin on his face was the best feeling ever. This was a MOMENT!

The point I'm trying to make is that despite all the twists and turns in life, we are now here. In this period of being able to share THE MOMENTS all the time. Our past was the road we had to travel in order to share the life we now have. It wasn't always easy, but it sure was worth it to share what we have now.

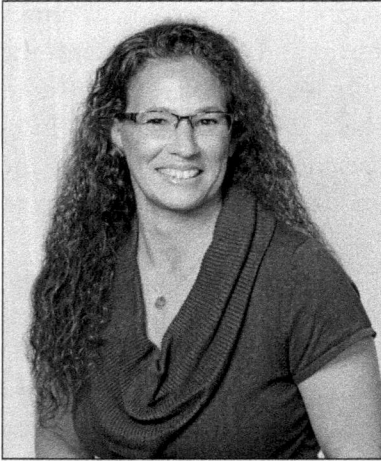

ABOUT MICHELLE PICKING

Michelle is a certified personal trainer, also holding certifications as a specialist in sports nutrition and strength and conditioning and is currently working on a menopause coaching certification. She's also a USA Weightlifting Level 1 Coach, a USA Weightlifting National Referee and currently holds all national records in the Master's Division W50–54, 64kg category.

Michelle started Rise Up Fitness to continue her love of helping people and creating a safe, judgment-free space for them to train, grow, and find new boundaries they choose. I believe in meeting clients where they are and helping them navigate the choices that lead them to a healthier lifestyle.

Michelle also decided to go back into her career as a veterinary technician/hospital manager and runs a veterinary surgical specialty practice. She uses her knowledge of how to grow to encourage her staff to continue their journey along the way as well.

To Connect with Michelle

Email: boothmichelles@aol.com
Facebook: @MichellePicking
Instagram: @michellepicking
Phone: 910-670-2759

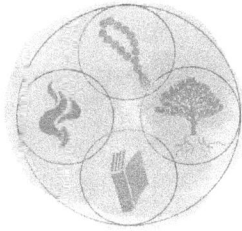

2022

Amber Whitt

After fighting my own self through hell and back, I've often wondered to myself, *Who else has walked through their own sort of hell and simply doesn't talk about it? Who else has survived their own torture and lived to tell the tale* . . .

I grew up in what you would call a normal, middle-class family. Both of my parents worked for themselves, and I strived to make them proud. I did my time for many years in the corporate world, and then I decided to venture out on my own and start my own business. I had my own company, but it was so hard in the beginning. We were broke, it was super challenging, but I wouldn't give it up. I'm stubborn as hell. I was determined to make it work. Finally, after years of hard work, it grew, and it grew so much and so well that my husband left his steady income job with amazing benefits to join me.

We were presented with an absolutely amazing business opportunity. We were going to be part of an up-and-coming massive franchise, but it was going to cost us a big chunk of money—money that we didn't have. We had just built our home that I manifested for years . . . We had only been living in our dream home for six months. Six figures and then some was the

73

buy-in cost. Ouch. I was about to leverage us on a lot of hopes and promises. I wasn't taking this decision lightly. After a lot of thoughts over it and "sleeping on it," I was all in. I had to have it. I convinced my husband that it would be an amazing opportunity, the growth process would be terrific, and this investment would be setting us up for retirement. It sounded almost too good to be true; so, we did our research, we believed in what we were being told, and we decided to move forward with full force! I'm stubborn like I mentioned, and if anyone was going to make this happen, I was bound and determined.

From the beginning, there were certain things and ways of doing business that I didn't completely understand and agree with, but this was coming from someone who had supposedly been doing this for many years, so I believed in him and the team. Every day I sat down and did the work; for two solid years, I gave every ounce of my being to this new business. Marketing, strategizing, helping others, building this business to the best of my ability, trainings, Zooms constantly, but the business itself couldn't grow and run properly or make money without the help and the hands of the other parts of the business. Those parts were completely out of my control. Things weren't moving forward as we were promised. Red flags were being thrown up all over the place, and I was starting to have my doubts about this new business venture. It felt like we were on a slowly sinking ship, and we needed to abort sooner than later. We weren't getting paid, there was no money coming in, and things were taking a turn for the worse. We decided it was in our best interest to opt out. No money was being returned to us, and no money that was owed to us for our sales was being paid.

My mental stability was on the line, and it shifted rather quickly. I remember the shift like it was yesterday. Out of nowhere, I was easily irritated, explosive with anger, and a rage and fire inside of me. I was taking it out not only on myself but on my beloved family. I was quick to lash out, yell, scream, throw myself on the ground, and during one of my few tantrums, I threw my phone across the room and my MacBook as well. This went on for many months. It was terrifying.

I was prescribed new medications by my doctor, and I was using all of the tools that I had in my tool set: meditation, working out, nature, breath work, and also working with my mentor weekly for energy work and discussions of what was happening. I was at a loss. I cried so much and for so long, I just wanted to feel better again and wanted hope and worthiness.

Nothing was helping me to get better, and my family was absolutely terrified of me. I could see it on their faces. I would walk into a room, they would look at each other, and no one knew who was walking in. I wasn't myself. I couldn't stand myself, so how could they? I wasn't me. I felt so chaotic every moment of every day; I kept asking, *Who am I? Why is this happening? Why can't I find myself? I am not me. How do I get back to me?*

I didn't want to die, but I didn't want to be with myself any longer. I seriously could not stand myself; I thought I was absolutely worthless, less than. I hated myself. I wanted to be ripped away from this earth, but not of my own fault. I was very fearful of what my next move was going to be toward myself, my family, my home; I was reckless. I was having a full-force mental breakdown, and the shift in my mental stability was so hard and happened so fast that I had no idea what I was supposed to do with myself—except lean on the tools that I have provided to myself and to others for many years as I had learned how to tend to my depression and my anxiety and all of the other disorders that I had been labeled with from a young age.

I reached out for help. I finally found a therapist who could see me in a short amount of time: a week and a half. Everyone else was on a six-month-plus waiting list, and I told them I couldn't wait that long. For my own sake, and my family's sake, I needed help, and I needed it now. I was scared, I was hopeless, I was terrified, and I was really ashamed. That new business venture was leaving us very far in debt, and I was extremely embarrassed and very ashamed of a business that was failing, but it wasn't failing because of my efforts. I had pushed, and I had pushed, and I had pushed so hard, but the business couldn't come to full fruition because we had been lied to and things weren't as they were supposed to be . . . A lot of smoke and mirrors.

I had to deal with that loss. I had to grieve it and deal with the embarrassment, but only of what I was telling myself. The shame I was feeling and tending to was put in my head by me, no one else. I had to actually come to terms with this by sitting with myself and knowing that I had done everything in my power to make the business come to full fruition, but sadly, I just couldn't.

I started therapy twice a week. I leaned on my mentor for spiritual help and guidance. I was open with everyone, and I felt so ashamed and unsettled. I remember my first therapy session; I could barely speak. The embarrassment, the reality of losing a major investment, feeling like I should've known better, but I had believed.

I needed space, and I needed a lot of it. I asked for it, and I was allowed a lot of downtime. I stepped away from our company to let my husband and our general manager run it. I sat in meditation for hours daily. The first few days I just sat and cried in my meditation room that my husband built and created for me, out of love and care. I had this beautiful space in our home to go to when I needed to escape. This was my space of solitude for an entire month, not just this room solely, but also my backyard, which is full of gorgeous, tall green trees, and bountiful grass to walk through and reconnect with nature.

During one of my lengthy meditations, I watched myself being reborn. I didn't understand what was happening at the time, but afterward, it was amazing to recap. As I was writing in my journal that I kept near me, it came to me, an understanding of what had just happened. A beautiful, bright white light and a baby coming down from the night sky, landing in the sand, and at the feet of people that were standing around a beautiful, tall, roaring fire. There was a Native American wearing a headdress with his feet dancing around in celebration of this new baby. It was a party, but I didn't understand it during my meditation; it was only when journaling after the fact, plain as day, that it was me being reborn. What a celebration indeed. I sobbed for hours. A new version of me had entered the world, and I felt the old version of me passing away in a sense, the version of me that hated myself, and that version that told me daily how much I was unworthy and how loathsome I was. That version was passing on, and I had a new outlook on myself, and life.

I stayed in therapy for a very long time. I didn't go quite as often any longer, and I shifted my appointments to a little farther out as I started getting better. I had found myself again, through meditation daily, major space, allowing myself to grieve and work through the loss of a major investment and what I thought of myself. Self-sabotage is a real thing, and our mind will tell us horrible thoughts that aren't really true. I learned how to balance my nervous system and to understand what is happening before I get too far into my self-talks of unworthiness or self-hatred. I'm not so hard on myself these days, and I offer myself a ton of grace and ease and a lot less judgment. Some days, that's a lot easier said than done.

I hope in whatever chaos or struggle you are facing that you know nothing lasts forever and to hold on very tightly as "this too shall pass."

I always knew how loved I was, especially during my struggles, as it was shown to me. We are never fighting these battles alone. Hang on for another day, even if it's just minute by minute, breath by breath, step by step.

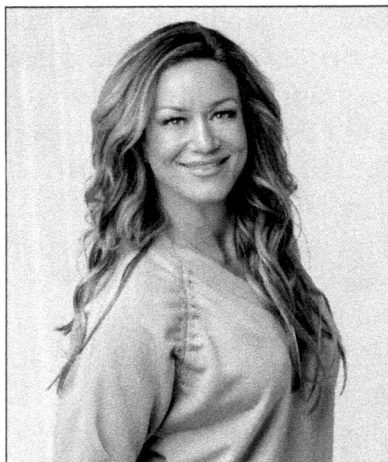

ABOUT AMBER WHITT

Amber owns multiple businesses as the creator and CEO. She has received several awards over the years for her excellence in business development, communication, marketing, strategizing, and sales.

Amber left the corporate world and started her residential cleaning company from the ground up in 2010, and it has grown exponentially. Amber not only helps her clients remove old energies and clear space from their homes, but also heals them personally and physically through her energy and sound healing practice, along with hosting retreats with her mentor.

Amber enjoys helping and supporting others all over the world in many ways, from distance reiki to sound healing, chakra cleansing, guided meditations, coaching sessions, and more. She believes wellness begins within oneself, and she has done a tremendous amount of inner work to help heal herself and to help guide others on their journey inward to self-discovery and awareness. She is always a work in progress, progress over perfection.

Amber loves to speak at intimate and larger events. Her enthusiastic approach to business, mental and physical health, life, and personal development makes her a wealth of knowledge on many levels. She's a highly motivated person who loves to dream big in all areas of her life.

To Connect with Amber

www.AmberWhitt.com

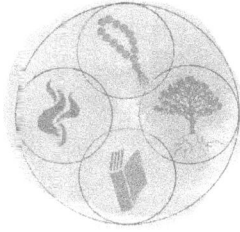

EMBRACING THE POWER OF
THIS PRESENT MOMENT

Tracey Watts Cirino

Hello, and welcome to the power of living in the present moment and creating moments that take your breath away. As I sit down to pour my heart into this chapter, I can't help but feel an overwhelming sense of gratitude for the chance to connect with you on a deep, meaningful level. You see, I'm not just a wife, mom, #1 best-selling author, or award-winning entrepreneur—I'm someone who has walked a path similar to yours, searching for the true meaning of happiness, success, and fulfillment.

I used to be caught up in the whirlwind of being a workaholic, believing that success meant sacrificing every precious moment with my loved ones. If I could just work a little harder, do more, I would finally be enough. But something inside me started tugging at my heartstrings, urging me to take a step back and reassess my priorities. Maybe you've felt that too—the yearning for a life that's more than just a series of checking off the overwhelming amount of boxes on your to-do list.

And here's the thing, my friend: I discovered that real freedom lies in creating a life that's aligned with your deepest desires and the moments that truly matter. It is about searching within instead of looking for pieces of significance outside of yourself. It's not about being overwhelmed and stressed out. It's about finding joy—not chasing balance, but discovering harmony and purpose every single day.

I get it, though. It can be a challenge to navigate the responsibilities we have to everything outside of ourselves: our kids, our husbands or partners, and our teams while still honoring ourselves and our dreams. But guess what? Today is the day that changes everything. Today, you're making a powerful decision—the decision to prioritize the moments that matter most to you over everything else.

So, as we embark on this incredible journey together, I want you to know that you're not alone. I've been in your shoes, grappling with the fear of letting others down, feeling like I was failing in every area and questioning whether it's even possible to break free from the status quo. Is this it? Does it get any better than this? The answer, my friend, it absolutely does when you make the decision to make the change.

Today, right here, in this very present moment, you have the opportunity to rewrite your story. It's time to let go of the past and step into a future that's bursting with possibility. No more settling for less than you deserve. No more putting your dreams on hold while you pretend everything is okay. Muttering under your breath I'm F-I-N-E. Today, you awaken as a new, empowered version of yourself, and there's no turning back.

I want you to know that the moments that matter—the ones that light up your soul and bring you pure joy—are waiting for you. They're not some distant dream; they're within your reach, my friend. All it takes is a simple decision—a decision to prioritize your well-being, your dreams, and your happiness. Your decision to decide right here and now to begin your journey of living a Beyond Common life that truly lights up your soul.

So, let's dive into the story filled with wisdom, practical tools, and inspiration to guide you on this incredible journey. Together, you will discover the secrets to breaking free from the common trap of being fine, embracing the power of the present moment, and designing a life that's authentically yours.

I'm beyond excited to walk alongside you as you embark on this life-changing adventure. Let's redefine success together, my friend, and create a life of freedom, purpose, and deep fulfillment. The moments that matter are calling your name, and I can't wait to witness the incredible transformation that awaits you. Here are a few of the best questions to ask to help you get started on revealing your best self.

Are you truly living your best life?

How often are you truly present?

What makes you laugh so hard your belly gets a workout?

What do you really want? If you are not sure here, go outside, take a walk, meditate, practice yoga, or do something creative you love to clear your head, and then ask again.

What do you really want? If you still need help going deeper with this to reveal what you really want grab my free clarity tool. https://www.beyondcommoncoaching.com/7layers

This is the Beyond Common 7 Layers deep process I use with my high level one on one clients to help them get unstuck so they can focus on what they really do want. It is a powerful tool to help you get the clarity you need.

The Power of Moments

As you embark on your quest to discover "Moments that Matter," I hope you can feel the energy of all the stories and the journeys of women who have dared to dream, shine, and embrace their worthiness. It is an honor to stand on the shoulders of these strong women as we all grow stronger together, to create a tapestry of inspiration and empowerment.

Before you dive into the depths of your moments.

Tell me, what are the moments that matter most to you?

What dreams have been quietly whispering in the depths of your soul?

What steps have you taken, or perhaps hesitated to take, toward designing a life that goes beyond mere checking boxes on your to-do lists?

Reflecting on the wisdom shared in *The Light That Shines Bright* and *Women Who Shine*, I am reminded of the brilliance that lies within every woman. It is a brilliance that radiates from a place of authenticity and self-love, illuminating the path to our true purpose. Now, imagine embracing those moments that ignite that light within you.

In *You Are Worthy* and *Women Who Dream*, we explored the power of self-belief and the transformation that unfolds when we recognize our inherent worthiness. Remember that you are deserving of every moment that sparks joy within you, fulfills your soul, and aligns with your core heart-centered values. It is time to claim your worthiness and step into the life you have always imagined.

And in *Dear Younger Self*, we introduced *You'll See* and we danced between the realms of innocence, worthiness and the confidence to follow your dreams, I offer reassurance and guidance. Your dreams are valid, no matter how audacious they may seem at the moment or to others. You have the power to shape your destiny, to create a life that harmonizes with the moments that truly matter to you. Embrace the lessons from the vantage point of "you'll see" when you encounter a nonbeliever and honor the journey that has brought you to this very moment.

"Becoming Beyond Common" holds the key to designing a life that revolves around the moments that matter most. It is a call to action, urging you to break free from societal expectations and chart a path that aligns with your true purpose and desires.

Together, we delve into the twelve essentials for success in life and the workplace, as revealed in *Beyond Common 12 Essentials for Success in Life and in the Workplace*.

As you work on creating more moments that matter in your daily life, open your heart to the possibility of living a life of fulfillment and purpose. Embrace the tools and insights shared, for they are the stepping-stones that will guide you toward your own Beyond Common journey. But remember inspiration without action is merely a flicker. It is time to ignite the flame of transformation within you.

So, I invite you to reach out and share your Beyond Common story with me. Let the words on these pages inspire you to take action, to create a ripple effect that will touch the lives of thousands of women around the world. Together, let us build a community of empowered female business owners who design their lives around the moments that truly matter.

The time has come to embrace them, step into the brilliance of your own light, and create a life that defies convention.

May this present moment be the catalyst for your own remarkable Beyond Common journey, where dreams are realized, your purpose is fulfilled, and the moments that matter become the foundation of your legacy.

As you turn the page, remember that you are worthy of every extraordinary moment that lies ahead. Let the power of your dreams and these stories, and tools ignite the fire within you and propel you toward a life that exceeds all expectations. That takes you far BEYOND what is Common so you can thrive. The world is waiting for you to unleash your brilliance and embrace *your moments that matter.*

With love and gratitude ♥,

Tracey Watts Cirino

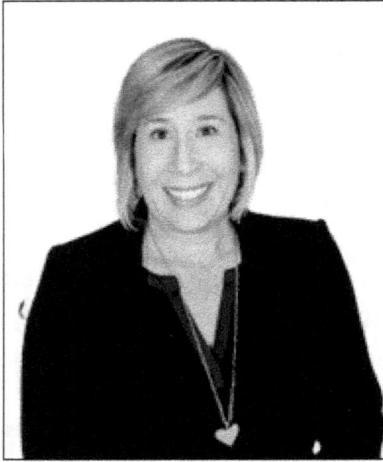

ABOUT TRACEY WATTS CIRINO

Tracey Watts Cirino is a five-time #1 International Best-selling author, award-winning business owner, highly engaging empowering speaker and podcast host of *Beyond Common Business Secrets* which is ranked in the top 5 percent of all podcasts.

Tracey is a powerhouse dedicated to helping entrepreneurs achieve greatness. With dynamic keynotes, transformative retreats, immersive workshops, digital training programs, and exclusive mastermind groups, she empowers business owners and leaders to harness their personal power and create customized success systems.

As the founder and CEO of Beyond Common Coaching & Consulting Company, a Cleveland, OH-based business that provides business growth strategies and speaking services to business owners across the world, Tracey is a Certified Success and Mindset Coach, Certified Canfield Success Principles Trainer, and John C. Maxwell certified speaker, coach, and trainer.

To learn more about how Tracey can help you achieve your personal and professional goals and to book Tracey as your speaker at your next virtual or in-person event, visit www.traceywattscirino.com.

To Connect with Tracey

www.TraceyWattsCirino.com
Facebook: Tracey Watts Cirino
Facebook Group: Beyond Common Women in Business Supportive Community
Instagram: @traceywattscirino
LinkedIn: Tracey Watts Cirino
YouTube: @traceywattscirino
Beyond Common Business Secrets Podcast:
https://podcasts.apple.com/us/podcast/
beyond-common-business-secrets/id1542242275

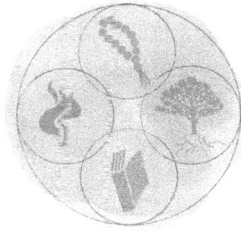

ADVERSITY TO OVERCOMING

Alexia Clonda

From an early age, I've been sick. I can't remember a time in my life when I've been a hundred percent well. Diagnosed with asthma and a heart murmur at only ten months of age, I was behind the eight ball from the very beginning. As a kid, I was always taking medicine—whether it be for asthma or an infection. It was always medicine, medicine, medicine.

Oddly, as I hated sports, when I was thirteen, a friend introduced me to squash. The local club manager spotted my talent and said to me, if you eat, breathe and live squash I will help you become a champion. I was hooked and how ironic.

Throughout my junior playing years, my asthma wasn't too bad. It was manageable, but I had it: it was clearly there. I also got serious bouts of pneumonia and, again, lots of infections. Just by having an infection, you're not at a hundred percent. Looking back at my career I reckon I was functioning between thirty and seventy percent most of the time. Then when the asthma worsened and became life-threatening, I had to use a nebulizer. I was nebulizing albuterol every four hours and always taking albuterol puffers, using up to five per month on top of the nebulizer. I carried a puffer everywhere; I could not leave home without it.

Then I was put on inhaled, oral (tablets) and IV corticosteroids. I was on an average dose of 30 milligrams of steroids per day for sixteen years. I was taking antibiotics every six weeks; it just went on and on and on. I was taking so many pills, I rattled. I wasn't well, and it was always at the back of my mind. But I never let it stop me from doing anything. I just found a way around it—not through it. Because I wanted to be the best squash player I could be and hated taking medication, I was always on the lookout for information and other ways to better manage the asthma.

I sought out a lot of alternative therapies after I was diagnosed with life-threatening asthma as my doctors said I would be on medications for the rest of my life. There was talk that I might grow out of it, but, as the years went by, I realized that wasn't going to happen. I wasn't going to grow out of it. It was with me as my cross to bear, so to speak. When the doctors told me I had to give up squash, as it could kill me, I remember making a decision. I would not let the asthma control me! So, with medication, I learned how to control it; but unfortunately, it did require a lot. There are the usual side effects; some didn't happen because I was extremely fit; but some did affect me, especially my muscles.

I couldn't retain muscle mass because corticosteroids waste muscle tissue. On my travels in the UK, one British Olympian doctor told me that it wouldn't be a bad idea to take a course of anabolic steroids just so I could retain some degree of muscle mass. I didn't do that and for the 9 years of my professional squash career, I traveled with a suitcase of medications and my nebulizer.

To add to the asthma, at twenty-six years of age, my spine developed disc protrusions. The sciatic nerve pain was going down both legs and the pain was excruciating. A spinal fusion was my only option. The doctor said that it could go one of three ways: (1) yep, you'll play squash again, not a problem, (2) You'll just be able to walk again with pain . . . maybe without some pain, or (3) You could end up in a wheelchair. Who knows? You might be a paraplegic. They wouldn't know until after the operation. I was only twenty-eight when I had to make the big decision to have the surgery. That was tough, but again, I took it in stride and thought, *well, what's meant to be is meant to be. I will do the best that I can do.*

At twenty-nine years of age, I had a spinal fusion. After the surgery, I had to lie on my back for a whole month in the hospital and relearn how to walk. I even had to learn how to get out of bed, sit, and get out of a chair. Walking was difficult. For the first six months after my operation, there was little communication between my brain and the bottom half of my body. I finally got on the court after six months. It was so frustrating: I would watch the ball but couldn't move.

I thought, oh no! This is it; my squash is over. But that inner voice kept saying, "don't give up, you can do this".

I had to adapt to the attitude of *okay, I'm going to beat this whatever happens. I'm going to do whatever I need to do, whatever it takes to get back on that court and lead the life I want to lead.* I always had to learn different ways to do things—not like the other squash players—but my way, so I could achieve what I desired. Sometimes it was very tough, and it wore me down physically and emotionally. I thought it would be easier just to give up, vegetate, and go through the motions of living; but because I still wanted to play squash and there was this something in the back of my mind, it was always my motivational force and inspiration. In 1991 I officially retired from the professional squash tour.

I still played squash as I loved it and I learnt that by being fit, I could tolerate more than most and I did not want to give up on me. However, I would get chronic fatigue and many more injuries, health and personal issues.

Somehow there was this strength, coming from somewhere that gave me my determination, tenacity, and grit to keep going. During the chronic fatigue period, it was painful to walk and even lift my head off the pillow. I remember taking some disgusting medications as an alternative therapy. My goodness, it tasted and smelled so bad.

There was always pain, and I was holding all that pain in. I did not let it out since I didn't want anyone to view me as weak. I thought vulnerability was a sign of weakness. It was fortunate that I learned to cry, to let it out, through the spiritual and self-development courses I became interested in after reading a spiritual healing book, You Can Heal your Body by Louise Hay in my early twenties. I wanted to learn how to communicate with myself, how to improve myself and I had this knowing that there was more to me than just squash.

I knew that I was resilient and strong, but I did not know how to access it, other than via squash. My determination to keep on playing and be a good squash player persisted . . . and because I liked it. I assumed there could be other ways to motivate myself. What were they? I thought spiritual healing would be a good way because believing in God or that higher power—that creator of energy, life force, creative intelligence, divine intelligence—whatever you want to call it, I knew was within me, and I was a part of it. The more I learned about it, the more I was open to learning more.

I realized that *hey, I am powerful. I know how to tap into and get into the flow of my own power to motivate me in kinder ways.* It was not to be through challenging ways—all the illness in my thirties, the chronic fatigue, more surgeries, stress fractures, and fasciotomies. Again, that was tough. Then in my late thirties and forties, I became fitter. I was starting to feel good. Despite being fit, I still had a compromised immune system. There were more illnesses—especially respiratory illnesses—and more injuries to my knees and hips.

My body was constantly in pain. I wasn't listening to my body, so it was constantly injured or in a state of illness. Through all the drugs and the wear and tear on my body, my immune system was telling me, "You're not helping me. You are hindering me with what you're doing. So, I'm going to weaken."

My asthma was well-managed by now, as I came across a breathing technique in 1994 when my asthma was at its worst. At the time, I was on 100 milligrams of steroids and nebulizing every hour. I thought I was going to die because no amount of medication was controlling the asthma. That's when I became fortunate. It was all over the news and in the media.

A breathing technique from Russia had landed in Australia. It was called the Buteyko Breathing Technique. I saw it on TV and in the newspapers. There were these free workshops, and Mum said, "Nothing to lose; you're not well, so give it a go."

I remember sitting at this workshop with my arms folded, thinking, *hang on, this is just too easy, and just too simple!* They were explaining to only breathe through your nose. I just went, *no, it can't be that simple. No doctor had ever told me this. No physiotherapist had ever told me this. This is just too simple.* I did the course over four days.

I was able, after months of practicing the breathing technique, to change my breathing and decrease the medications I was on. This helped me get back into squash.

This breathing technique was a life changer and saver. I got fitter and stronger in my forties and started to play in tournaments again. In 2007, at the age of 46, I played the Australian Closed Championship, along with quite a few other tournaments. I was beating a couple of the top twenty players in Australia. All these players were half my age, they couldn't work out how I was beating them. It was because I had the experience and the knowledge. I also had grit and determination, part of that never-give-up attitude.

With the breathing, I realized that I had more control over my health and body than I had thought. This was mind opening. I began to teach it—which was even better—to help another person realize that they have the power to change their circumstances, control and change them to be empowered and create their own circumstances.

This has fascinated me ever since. I keep doing it because I always thought asthma was there to help me assist other people to prove that no matter what you're going through—no matter what illness or injury and whatever life throws at you—you are creating your own reality. Life doesn't happen to you; it's happening for you.

Throughout childhood, you've been programmed with certain beliefs. I recognize now that these beliefs really have held me back. It was through asthma and illnesses—and pretty much from my fifties onward—that I came to see this reality more and more. Again, it was through spiritual teachings that I've learned that the outside reflects what is inside. We can change what's within us: our feelings, our thoughts, and our self-talk. I also learned that with squash, you've got to think positively and believe in yourself. You need to engage in positive self-talk, be your own best friend.

In my fifties, I got even more into spirituality, in particular ThetaHealing®. I realized that I have the power to create my own reality. I changed my beliefs, how I spoke to myself, and what I thought. Negative thoughts still come up, but you don›t have to accept them. You can change them by asking yourself the question, "What›s this really about, what's this teaching me?" A great example of this is when I lose a match. I ask myself, "What could I have done better? What could I have changed? What am I learning from this?" They're the same questions you can ask in your life. "What am I learning from this situation, this experience?"

People trigger us all the time—especially our families and friends. That trigger is an opportunity to help you learn and grow . . . and to expand and evolve. Ask yourself the appropriate questions: "What's this teaching me? What can I learn from this? What do I need to learn from this?" It's about being open to unlearning the old assumptions. It's about changing former beliefs, recognizing that those you grew up with, what you formulate, or what your mind was programmed to believe—are all changeable.

As an adult, you recognize that they're hindering you, holding you back, and you can change them. It's about recognizing and identifying those beliefs first, then replacing them with beliefs that are empowering and positive to help you expand and grow.

This really rang true when I developed anxiety, going through a rough time at work. I was the CEO of a sporting association, and it was very stressful. I was diagnosed with PTSD, developed from that position. I was overcome with self-doubt, about my own capabilities because I wasn't a professional squash player anymore, I was in the administrative world now, i.e., the corporate world. There were a lot of expectations of me, and a lot of people's opinions weren't all positive. I was being bullied and sexually harassed. It wasn't just coming at me from one direction: it was coming from all directions. I felt betrayed and struggled to trust people because even though I was getting good results I had people attacking me, which confused me.

I started to doubt myself and everything I did. The process wears you down emotionally, spiritually, physically, and mentally. When you hear people put you down—saying things that are not true and lying about you—you start to believe it. You start to think: *What am I doing here? What's the purpose of my life? If I'm not helping or improving things or doing good things, why am I here? And why is all this stuff happening to me? I'm not a bad person.*

Self-doubt is like an anchor; it weighs you down. I began to think, *What's the point of being here when all this illness, and these injuries, keep pulling me down?* I would take a couple of steps forward and then huge steps backward. It's like I couldn't get a break. I wanted to end it all numerous times, but for some reason, at the back of my mind, there was this voice that insisted, "No, you're here to do something; you're here to do something." So, I just kept hanging in there.

What am I here to do? was the big question. My answer has been here the whole time: helping other people. I had been a strong supporter and volunteer for the Australian Lung Foundation and the New South Wales Asthma Foundations. I helped people understand how to not let their illness control them, letting them know that whatever they were experiencing, they could get through it. The guiding force in the back of my mind in my energy field was and is, *I can get through it.*

As I get older, it's becoming clear that if I can just help one other person not go through what I've gone through or understand that they can change it, I'll know I have made a difference. My life purpose is contributing to a greater good—a greater purpose. Whatever anyone is going through, they can get over that mountain, that hurdle. No matter what mountain is put in front of them, they can climb over it and get to the other side. My role in life is to uplift people and help them to understand themselves—in short, to ignite that fire within.

We all have a fire within ourselves. I think my role in life is to help inspire and reignite—that fire within each person I encounter. I'm here to help them reconnect with themselves so they can remember that they are empowered to create their own reality and live the life of their dreams. Discovering that whatever we think is a challenge, we can turn it around, reframe it into an opportunity and become aware of the infinite possibilities around us to be who we truly are, sparks of love.

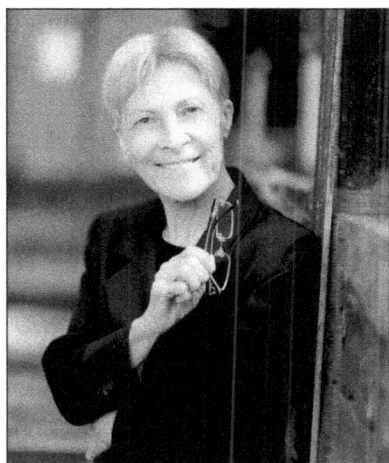

ABOUT ALEXIA CLONDA

Meet Alexia Clonda, an outlier in adversity. She is a luminary in the fields of breathing, mindset, and spiritual coaching, and an exceptional high-performance squash coach. Born into a life of adversity, she was beset by chronic asthma and an initial disdain for sports as a result. It was painful to exert herself physically, as the asthma worsened.

Alexia's tale is not one of comfort but of continuous challenge and relentless determination. Despite these obstacles, she blossomed into the number one junior squash player in the world. Then in adulthood despite life-threatening asthma, she became one of the best players in the world, with a world ranking of number five.

Alexia embodies resilience and tenacity. Her life thus serves as a powerful testament to the human spirit and the ability to achieve the seemingly impossible. Her ability to turn adversity into a catalyst for transformative change has led her on a personal path to help others. As a breathing, mindset, and spiritual coach, Alexia is a guide to unlocking the full potential within, empowering people to uncover their innate capabilities, thereby enhancing every aspect of their lives. This holistic approach, encompassing the mind, body, emotions, and soul guarantees transformation.

Connect with Alexia:

Web: www.themindbreathingedge.com
Email: mindbreathingedge@gmail.com
Web: www.alexiaclonda.com

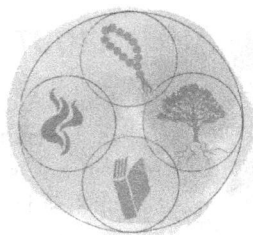

HONORING THE MOMENT

Jennifer Eaker

The Power of a Moment
As we pass by one another, life going around us,
How do we slow it down and let it just be?
A smile, a hug, the heartbeat between two, memories being made,
Brings a moment in the making.
Life is a collection of moments that embraces the beauty . . .
Beauty of love shared, opened opportunities that come along your way,
Lessons learned, friendship and a reflection of what's to come.
We remember the moments that are experienced and shared.
Something simple as a hug, smile, helping one another,
Can bring meaning and influence on one's day.
Intentional interactions, purpose and impact brings power to the moment.

Throughout the years, I have had opportunities to have some beautiful memories with family and friends. However, in those moments, I always thought there would be one more concert, one more time celebrating a friend's birthday, one more time for anything and everything. Even though in my head I knew the saying, "Life is short," in those moments, when hanging out with family or friends, I just would not think of that, or maybe I just didn't want to believe that it could be all gone within a blink of an eye.

It took the loss of a friend to impact me and open my eyes to see the power in a moment that I could have between my interactions with people. I really appreciate the moments being made and how it's important to honor these moments with whom that have passed on. What follows is my story of losing a friend and how it impacted me. I hope you will find inspiration in this story; may it bring some type of healing for those who have lost someone and help people truly appreciate the beauty of the various moments in their life.

I was at home ten years ago when I found out the news. The news that my friend's, who was in law enforcement, life ended in the line of duty. I instantly felt like someone just punched me where it was hard to breathe. I was gasping for air, overwhelmed by the feelings that just flooded me. How was this even possible? I kept saying, "This can't be."

It had been a few years since we last saw each other, since I moved to another location. He was "good people," a great friend, loved his family, loved his job and serving the community. His life was taken by another's hand. Wrapping my head around the idea that someone ended my friend's life, I asked God why this would happen. My world seemed to be turned upside down, and I wasn't even part of his family. Anyone who knows me knows how I love all the people in my life no matter how long I have known you. My heart went out to his family and his coworkers (brothers/sisters in blue, his additional family), and I was just numb.

His death impacted me so greatly. There were days when I went through the motions because life continued, and I still had to work. There were days even surrounded by family and friends when I felt I just had no words. But the faith where I questioned God was the same faith where I leaned in more. As people around me found out that I just lost a friend, I heard, "Sorry for your loss." During this time of grief, hearing those words struck a nerve in me even though I knew people meant well by saying it. It's always hard to decide what to say to someone who is grieving, but it seemed like those words were what people instinctively said. This was one of the things I started changing in the upcoming years: changing the words said to make people feel more recognized, seen, and loved while in their grief.

I only knew my friend for a brief time compared to the time his family knew him or even compared to a lifetime. However, the memories we did share made me realize it's the moments we have with other people that they will be remembered by. You don't realize the power a moment holds until after the fact. It's important to acknowledge the moment, embrace it, treasure it, and find a way to share it with others.

After the death of my friend, I intentionally started taking even more pictures of everything and appreciating the memories being made between me and family and friends with more gratitude knowing that it could be gone all in a blink of an eye. It took this time to make me realize that life is precious, and I strive to value all kinds of moments in my life that are good and not so good. The word treasured has meaning to me, and I get to apply it to the people in my life and the moments shared.

In order to acknowledge and reflect on the shoes one has walked in, it's important to show honor by taking pieces of the memories shared to inspire and impact another. It took me what seemed like a long time to heal from the death of my friend. While questioning God about how this could happen, I also thought, How can I celebrate his life and the impact he had on others? So, every year after that, I intentionally do something to celebrate and honor his life on the day he passed away, and on his birthday, I honor him and the life that he carried. Doing this has also helped me through the losses of a few close people within the past ten years. It's helped me in a way to prepare me for these losses. I find ways to celebrate their life and memories we shared. I have learned the grieving process is different for each person that passed on and for the person grieving, but it has somewhat made the grieving process a little easier knowing I can celebrate their life by the moments we shared and then sharing them with others to help impact those more positively.

How Do You Want to be Remembered By?

Blue skies above, an array of colors ahead
Brings forth the interaction between the two.
Initiated conversations which leads to additional conversations continue . . .
In a room filled with many,
Smiles, hugs and laughter fill the air and are exchanged.
Sitting around the table among food that is savored,
Leads to a memory being made.
My feet feeling the sand between my toes,
Waves crashing, the sound of the ocean all around
Time spent with one another in conversation and the collection of seashells.
You walk in a room and the darkness turns to light.
How you just make everyone around you feel loved and seen,
The sparkle in your eye, the way you make people laugh brings a smile to other's faces.
When loneliness creeps in, to be that friend for another that you would want someone to be for you.
How you impact others to make a difference in their lives and the lives of others
It's in the moments that are intertwined with each of us, holding the capability of such power.
On this day, what will you do and decide, on how you want to be remembered by?

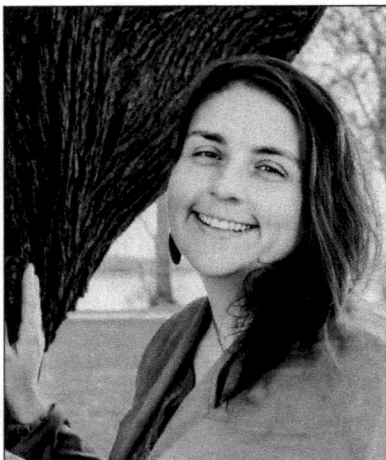

ABOUT JENNIFER EAKER

Jennifer is a writer, a creative spark for others, one who strives to inspire and impact.

She also dedicates some of her time as a Certified Oola Life Coach and Ambassador. For more information on that, you can visit this site: https://myoola.oolalife.com/JennEaker.

Oola focuses on finding balance, purpose, and growth in the seven key areas of life: fitness, finance, family, field, faith, friends, and fun.

Jennifer has loved writing poetry for several years, and one of her visions is for someone to be empowered and inspired to be the best they can be in all key areas of life, finding their voice within themselves to inspire another through experiencing poetic word. This is one of the first times she is sharing her work in a publication.

By sharing this story, she hopes people will appreciate life's moments as precious no matter how big, small, amazing, or not so amazing it is as well as find gratitude and a way to honor those moments.

To Connect with Jennifer

beyouwithoola@yahoo.com

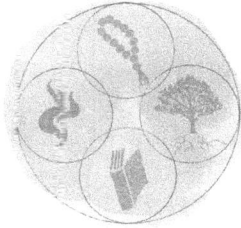

MONARCHS, MAGIC, & ME

Ann Marie Gill

When I least expected it, an unimaginable adventure began to unfold. In February 2017, I visited the Michoacan region of Mexico. It was the start of a special connection with me and the Monarch butterfly. Seeing the golden winged beauties at the overwintering grounds, I marveled that they had traveled over 4,000 km from my home in Ontario to the forests in Mexico, braving inclement weather and avoiding predators. I learned that these migrators are 4th generation monarchs, that live 6 to 9 months and are guided solely by instinct, an internal GPS.

On horseback at the first sanctuary, I awaited my group of fellow Canadian travelers to gather. The locals motioned me over to their resting space. In a hidden area, they pointed to a spot on the ground, a large, dark mud puddle. As I approached the puddle, it started to move. Dense clumps of butterflies were resting in the brown mud. I sat down to watch them, and waves of monarchs fluttered around me. Tears trickled down my face as I drank in the moment silently. Later, I discovered that these monarchs were male and were drinking in nutrients and minerals from the earth, a phenomenon called "puddling."

As I ventured up the mountain side, it was cooler in the

forest. I gingerly walked along the forest floor, careful not to step on monarchs that lay scattered on the ground. In the trees, they clustered together in roosts to stay warm, draping over branches like giant oversized pine cones. Hints of brown and shimmering orange revealed like enormous fall leaves on the trees. As the sun warmed, the sky filled with orange and gold. They gracefully soared and fluttered overhead, the soft sound of their wings like rustling tissue paper. When I closed my eyes, I could sense their gentle presence. So peaceful. Approaching one on a leaf, I was able to gently put my nose on its wings. We shared a moment of connection. The local guide on our trip was amazed to see the photo of my nose touching the butterfly wings. Was it a butterfly kiss? I felt a warm glow from this special moment.

Transformation

I grow milkweed in my garden, as it is the only food source for the caterpillars. My garden also has flowers for butterflies to nectar on, including native species. After witnessing several caterpillars being attacked, I realized how vulnerable they are, and it motivated me to start raising them. In the wild only one or two percent make it from egg to butterfly. The tiny egg transforms into a yellow striped caterpillar, and I nurture it through five stages of growth, feeding milkweed. The caterpillar then hangs upside down in a "J," its antenna drooping. It releases a green gooey substance and starts to spin its chrysalis as it wriggles and eventually sheds its outer skin. Inside the chrysalis, the muscles and organs dissolve and imaginal cells create a new form—the body and wings of the butterfly. I share my love for musical expression by singing and playing instruments for them throughout their development.

If someone told you that playing a musical instrument would influence the way a caterpillar formed its chrysalis, would you believe them? I'm not sure I would, but I witnessed it when I played my flute to a newly forming chrysalis. My caterpillar was halfway through metamorphosis, hanging upside down and enveloping its lower half with a green jelly-like substance to form its new home. As I played faster and louder, its body swayed quickly to the tempo and the green liquid released more rapidly. When I slowed the speed and lowered the volume, the green jelly slowed in production and the half chrysalis moved slowly, becoming more still. I was amazed, it was as if I was a conducting maestro. I continued to play my flute with a more tranquil quality, the music creating a soft backdrop for the dramatic process of change. From its silk tether, a jade and gold chrysalis gradually revealed itself as a beautiful jewel.

When the chrysalis changes color, the golden wings start to become visible. I sing and greet them as they enter the world in their new form of gold. At first the monarchs are plump, and their wings are short, like they are wearing a full ruffled skirt. I watch as they gracefully sway side to side. In their dance, their wings unfold and grow long. Feeling the transformational energy as I witness them shape shift from egg to caterpillar to butterfly never grows old. Each birth is unique and new, it is inspiring and magical.

After being in a car accident, I experienced a concussion for the first time in my life. Being surrounded by the transformational energy was a balm for me. I slowed down and went into my own chrysalis, enveloped in a darkened, quiet place of self-acceptance and healing energy.

I too can transform, to release things that do not serve me and become a new version of me. I can cast off my protective shell and go inwards to a safe space, a darkened space where I examine my inner reflections and release anything weighing me down. My own 'imaginal cells' can rearrange and align as I experience my own journey of healing and transformation. Witnessing the metamorphosis, a shape shift from egg to golden transformation, is an inspiration and example to me of the miraculous, of what is possible.

Milagro

Milagro, Spanish for "miracle," was the first butterfly I raised, a male. My tour guide in Mexico encouraged me to take a caterpillar I found in my garden and raise it. At that time, one of my dogs,

Tuffy was in the hospital with congestive heart failure. It was very stressful. I sent Tuffy energy healing and cared for the newly found caterpillar, feeding it milkweed, and cleaning its living space each day. The veterinarians did not think Tuffy was going to make it. I continued sending him distance healing and love, telling him to stay calm and to fight. Against all odds, and to the doctors' surprise, Tuffy was able to breathe on his own. Days later his kidneys were in crisis due to the diuretic medication. I continued to pray and provide energy healing and his kidneys improved. He was able to come home and be with his two brothers, which truly was a miracle! I still remember our car ride home. Tuffy solidly stood on the car seat as Elton John's "I'm Still Standing" played on the radio. Watching the chrysalis form was mesmerizing, another miracle. When the butterfly emerged, a local expert told me how to feed him and offered to tag Milagro for Mexico. I eagerly accepted and we met at a beautiful garden along the migratory route, called Rosetta McClain Gardens. When I released Milagro, he stayed nectaring on the flowers. Saying goodbye, I touched my nose to his wings and spoke to him about the beauty and the miracle he had shown me. With gratefulness in my heart, I thanked him for sharing part of his journey with me. I asked if he would like to go to Sierra Chincua, a beautiful sanctuary in Mexico, and his wings fluttered rapidly as if he understood me. Then he flew up and over the trees towards the lake.

Milagro's tag, number 649, was the last tag out of 1500 and saved for him. When I say the number 649 in Ontario, Canada, it is perceived as being lucky because it conjures up a vision of winning the lottery, Lotto 649. I knew I had already won the lottery. The winnings were not monetary but rather a wealth of magical experiences, of connecting my essence with a beautiful butterfly, the Monarch.

Second Chances

I joined the "tagging team" at Rosetta McClain. As citizen scientists we provide data on migrating butterflies to the University of Kansas.

One day at the gardens a little voice called out to me. "Miss, can you please help me," the young girl asked. She tugged on my hand and led me towards a flowering shrub. "This butterfly is injured and it can't fly. I have hidden it so the birds cannot get it." Although I had done energy healing on animals and insects before, this was my first venture into butterfly wing repair. I was nervous about the delicate procedure . . . secure the butterfly gently, keep the room dim and repair the wing with contact cement glue. Lightly brush talcum powder on the repaired wing seam, so that it would not stick to the surface below. After performing the repair, the butterfly rested. I put it on a flower and gave it energy healing. I held my breath in anticipation, "will it fly"? It flew high up into the trees. What a feeling, my heart soared!

Since then, I have been asked to assist with helping butterflies who are injured and cannot fly. The wing repairs are varied. Some involve putting a splint on a torn wing while others involve adding a piece of butterfly wing onto the existing wing. Sometimes when I release the repaired butterfly it flies gracefully into my garden or into the trees. Sometimes it takes to the sky and soars away. Each time I feel elated, filled with relief, wonder, and gratitude. It is a blessing to see them fly again, a reminder that second chances exist for all of us. Knowing this, life is full of promise.

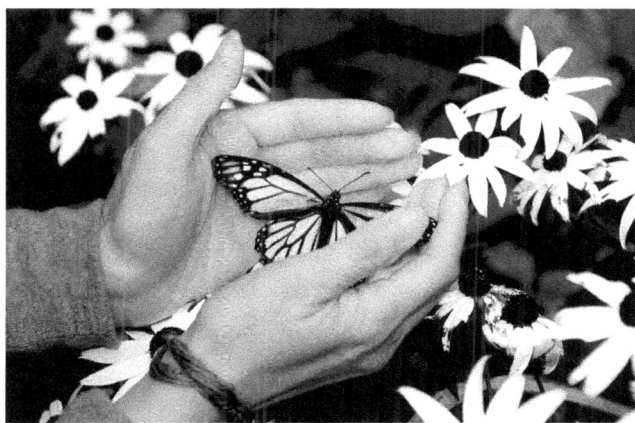

Olivia Lucy

Just as in life, sometimes the wing repair does not take. A butterfly named Olivia Lucy beat her wings strongly after repair but could not fly. The wing attachment broke. I performed two more repairs but it was not meant to be. She flapped her wings awkwardly and could not stay airborne. I felt frustrated for her and kept her comfortable, bringing her into the sunny garden for hours at a time, keeping a watchful eye on her. She really seemed to enjoy music, as I played instruments and sang. Once she even stayed on my shoulder and listened to the piano music for a long stretch. It had a calming effect on her. On the night she was transitioning, she perched on a flower bouquet of zinnias on top of my piano. I played and sang to her, then put her on my bedside table so she would not be alone. When I awoke in the morning she had fallen off the flowers and had passed away. Later that evening I briefly nodded off twice. Both times I had a dreamlike vision of her. She was in a forest, in a green tree—vibrant and full of life. The colors were vivid—like technicolor. I had seen her in my mind's eye. The woman who had raised her contacted me and gave me details about Olivia Lucy. It was then that I realized a thread of connection had woven this butterfly and I together. Olivia Lucy's birthday was October 10th, the same as mine!

Letting Go

I always have mixed emotions when it is time to release the monarchs. Letting go is difficult for me. I get 'butterflies' in my stomach. I have done all I can do, and now our journeys are taking different paths to fulfill our own individual destinies. I look for the best weather conditions, and with a lump in my throat and a song in my heart, I sing them a prayer for their journey. They have always let me close to them, allowing me to put my nose onto their wings if they are perched on a flower. To my surprise, some have alighted onto my face. Their little ambles on my face are softly ticklish. They have stayed with me for quite some time, taking in the music and saying a much-appreciated goodbye. I am filled with wonderment as time stands still. It is a release for me as well when they take flight. Sometimes I laugh, sometimes I cry. I feel a rush of energy and an accompanying sense of weightlessness. I am one with them.

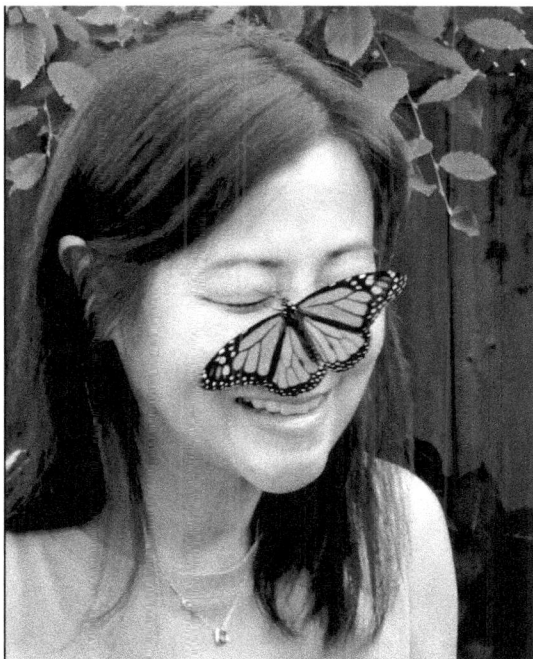

Fernando

One of my tagged butterflies was found. I released Fernando, the male butterfly, on September 1st. The notes from the finder said that Fernando was at "The Grand Hotel in Point Clear, Alabama with hundreds of other migrants. Caught it while tagging other monarchs." I got goosebumps! In 40 days, Fernando had traveled 2000 km, he was halfway to Mexico with friends! The song "Fernando" by Abba was playing in my head. I looked up the meaning of the song, and it is about two Mexican freedom fighters and liberation. Fernando was found on October 10th, my birthday, a sign from the Universe that what I was doing had meaning and purpose.

Liberation and The Journey Home

After leaving my corporate role I felt drawn to give back to the business world I was so familiar with. I was a certified yoga teacher and practitioner of meditation, Qigong, Tai Chi, and energy and sound healing. I knew that I benefited from self-care practices and it was sorely needed in the corporate setting. Once during a sales presentation, a client had a meltdown. He felt he was targeted by a new boss and as a single parent, feared losing his job. He began to cry and have a panic attack. I quietly asked him if he would like to try an exercise with me. He nodded yes. I started to lead him into breathwork, and he began to breathe more slowly and evenly. He quickly regained his composure and thanked me.

My first corporate wellness session was for a conference in Ontario. I was nervous and excited. In the morning I led a wellness session for financial advisors who were previously my clients. In the afternoon, I taught a customized session to a group of wholesalers. It was strange and exhilarating to meet fellow colleagues as a new me; not as a sales consultant but as a wellness consultant. I had shape shifted! Sharing techniques and witnessing participants' transformation was immensely fulfilling. Upon exiting the room I noticed a large banner and couldn't believe my eyes! Overhead, there was a monarch flying over a road, with the words: "Further, Faster, Liberation."

The theme of liberation was front and center. I pondered liberation, freedom and what it meant to me.

Just as the Monarchs use intuition to guide them home to Mexico, I feel guided. Whether it be nestled in a forest filled with butterflies, or a place in my heart where I can touch down and know that I am whole and complete, I am home where there is an unlimited reserve of unconditional love and acceptance.

The word "svatantrya" in the Tantric philosophy means "the freedom to be who you are." After holding myself back and staying in my protective chrysalis, I have been emerging to reveal some of the hidden me, finding my voice and being my authentic self by sharing my own unique expression in the world.

Through many forms of self-care, I am the best version of me. I have found a new voice in my singing, a deeper meaning in my martial arts and in the way I express myself as a creative. I am more present and mindful, letting go of my inner critic. I release things that throw me off balance with greater ease and accept things as they are.

The magical connection to the Monarch that started in Mexico has now expanded. I feel part of something bigger. Even when the butterflies are not physically with me, their essence and energy remain with me always. We are connected. I feel so blessed. They have brought me out of my chrysalis to share beauty and wonder. Synchronicities have been confirmations that I am on the right path. I stay open and connect to a bigger energy. I embrace the freedom to be who I am and journey into my heart where unconditional love, acceptance, and freedom are my birthright, a universal birthright for all of us.

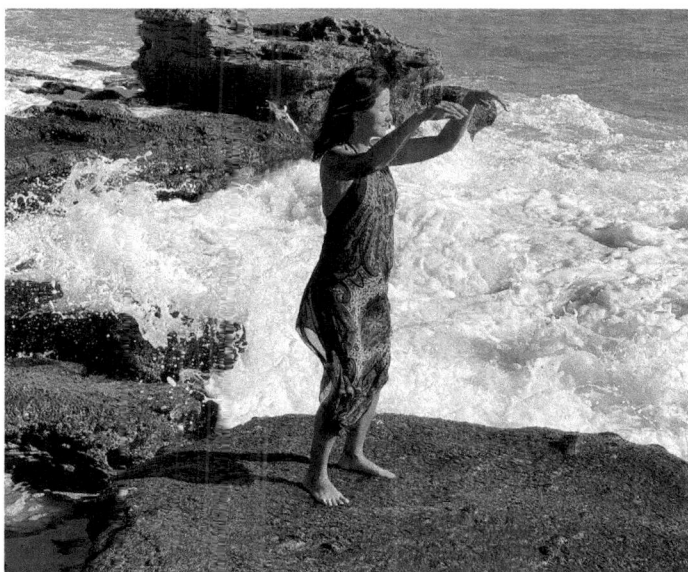

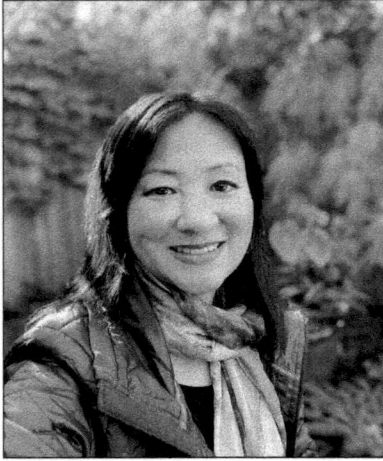

ABOUT ANN MARIE GILL

Ann Marie Gill is on a journey of self discovery. She follows her heart and sees signs and connections that guide her through life. She is open, inquisitive and loves to be in nature, where she finds peace and contentment.

An artist at heart, she loves to create, engaging in self expression through movement, music, and artistic endeavors. Since the age of 5, she has been singing and playing piano. Music is a gift to her soul. She cares deeply for the natural world and has been called a Monarch Whisperer.

Ann Marie is a Wellness Consultant, dedicated to inspiring positive transformational change in individuals. Having worked in multinational corporations, she understands the challenges and demands of the business world and enjoys sharing her learnings in the corporate setting. She is passionate about self care and educating with simple and effective tools for mind, body and spiritual wellness. She draws on knowledge from her certifications in yoga, sound therapy, energy healing, and practices of meditation, Tai Chi, Qigong, and kung fu.

To connect, book a speaking engagement or wellness event, please contact her at

amgdragonfly@gmail.com

Photo Credits:
Energy Healing—Rebekah Bennett
Butterfly on Face—Ken Yip-Chuck
Lift Water—Ken Yip-Chuck

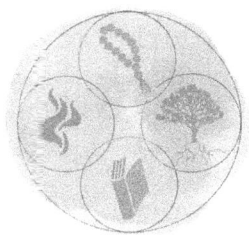

JUST KEEP MOVING

Nicole Smith Levay

I was four years old when I suffered the trauma that would forever change my life. My family and I were in our golden-beige minivan on our way to my cousin's Christening. There was broccoli salad in a tray lying on the floor between the seats up front. My father was driving, little brother was in a booster seat to my left, and my mother was in front of me. We were going up a winding hill on a rural road in New Jersey.

Then, it happened.

We crashed.

While I was too little to understand what happened or for my memory to store the details for years to come, I do remember, somatically, the moments before impact. The car screeched and spun slightly, the glass window shattered and sprinkled inside the vehicle. I can feel this in my guts, my lower back, as a picture comes to mind: my mother averting her face and lifting her arms. There is broccoli salad in the air. There is no sound and I can't see what happens next.

Many years later, after sorting through various conversations, I uncovered what really happened. The other driver coming down the hill was in our lane, so my father had to make a quick decision:

Turn the car off the hill into the trees or turn into the lane the oncoming car was supposed to be in? He chose the latter. He spun the wheel to the left but, in a split second, the other driver corrected his trajectory and moved to the same lane. It was too late to prevent tragedy from happening. The other driver crashed into my door. The impact sent us into the trees.

The next thing I remember is that I'm being cradled in my grandmother's arms. She is running with me toward a house and there is a lot of blood. I am choked for air, unable to make a sound. Eventually it comes, hard and slow, like a roar that shakes my soul. I cry a lot, echoing everybody else's cries as they lay me on a kitchen island or table. There is a light and I look up. In that moment, both the pain and the memory fade away. After that, only fragments: the ambulance, the hospital, an enormous cast on my right leg, my welcome home party with Cookie Monster.

Then, life went on. There was no talk about it in my conscious memories. For twenty-eight years, nobody spoke about it. Until I could no longer stand the silence. Or, my body began screaming at me, forcing me to break the silence. The expression "the body keeps the score" is true. As I write this for the first time, I can't feel my body. Trauma has a way of residing within you forever if you never confront and treat it.

What is trauma? How does it affect us and how does it ripple through the rest of our adulthood? Whether consciously or unconsciously, we tend to live our past.

When discussing trauma, I now know we are first and foremost speaking about the nervous system's response to an event, versus an actual event that happened. Trauma is subjective: the body system reacts in a fight, flight, freeze, or fawn state because our electrical current—our nervous system energy—says: "TOO MUCH TOO FAST, MAKE IT STOP!" Then the body and mind come up with clever ways to do exactly that:

1. Fight: lash out and project onto others, literally engage the body in aggression
2. Flight: disassociate or "leave" your body by spacing or numbing out
3. Freeze: breath is held, a shock that lasts a long while
4. Fawn: goes into caretaking others, dismissing one's own needs

These are the basics of trauma-sensitive healing. While intentions may be good, hurt people hurt people. Without knowledge of our own trauma and how it results in our body, we are primed to cause more harm in the world by enacting our trauma responses onto interpersonal situations, and not seeing others clearly. This in turn creates more pain for the traumatized individual, as they lose the ability to soothe themselves in relationships—known as coregulation. Being able to be soothed in relationship is a primary function in the wellness of human beings! When we know our own somatic trauma reactions, we can change our own lives and positively impact those around us.

Trauma takes on a life of its own. What is overwhelming to the system becomes split off and fragmented into emotions, images, thoughts, and physical sensations that intrude into the present until resolved. How could I possibly assume to know what's right around the corner at all times? Even if my mind told me I couldn't, I felt my body fantasize that it could. Hypervigilance had become my norm.

An armoring in my muscles, tensing within my joints, and a static and charged energy around the perimeter of my body. Aura small, eyes wide, eyebrows lifted. Body bolted by the worries and fears of the pain maybe to come.

Be afraid of what might happen, that'll help just in case, I told myself. *Brace for that impact, from any angle.*

Even with all that hyper-alertness, the traumatic pattern

repeated itself. It was as if it was written on me: *let the crisis come to me, I will handle it.* A little girl carrying so much emotional responsibility. Where does the heaviness go when it can no longer be held?

From age five to twenty-two, I danced two to eight hours a day, at least five or six days a week. I had chronic back pain ever since. Even now, after endless treatments and therapy, I experience issues in my spine occasionally. When I first started physical therapy, hunched over like an old woman wincing in pain, people would panic seeing such an unfamiliar site and awkwardly ask: "How could such a young woman hurt her back so badly? It's just not right!" I felt I needed to answer them, but had no idea. Someone did know the answer, *I just didn't know yet.* It wasn't even that I was too young to remember what happened, but I had blacked out during the most significant accident in my life.

At the time of my first bouts of chronic pain I was a young professional dancer, working hard. I blamed myself for a lack of awareness, not enough stretching, bad diet, or something else. Trauma has a way of making us feel like we are not enough and that everything is our fault. It robs us of our inherent lifeforce power, and leaves us riddled in fear, inner conflict, and lack of trust in what we perceive.

Years after repeated injuries, a doctor finally noticed that my right leg was significantly shorter than my left, a bit more than a half of an inch. How did this happen? This was not hip displacement, or caused by stress. The bones were different lengths. I didn't know what to say when people asked how I hurt myself. I remembered there was mention of a car accident a few times from family members. I had those snippets of flashback memories of something that seemed significant. There was a check from someone in that car accident that helped me pay for both continuing education and life expenses in my late twenties. I had seen photos of me with a cast, but didn't know anything else about the accident. That was it. We didn't talk about it in our house.

Twenty-four years after the car accident, I learned I had a physiological disability I didn't know about. My leg length discrepancy resulted in severe herniations in several vertebrae in my spine because of all of the asymmetric high intensity training through the years, unevenly compressing the discs. This meant a continuation of costly health care bills, and more painfully, I was told by multiple doctors that I would also need to transition out of my dancing career. This idea was traumatizing to my sense of self and my identity. There was also the physical trauma of not being able to walk, regular debilitating spine pain, and blacking out. All of the senses firing DANGER—ears ringing, seeing spots, hallucinations, full body migraines, being so dizzy I felt I could literally leave my body and disappear. I experienced these symptoms regularly. Not to mention the utter endless pain of grief in losing a piece of my soul as a dancer, never to be the same. It is still a daily practice of letting go of a life I embodied that I physically do not and will not have access to (at least in that way) ever again. Going from someone who felt at times like a superhuman athlete of God, spinning in multiple circles up on their toes, jumping six feet in the air, lifting other bodies upon their own, to someone who lives with chronic pain and needs customized orthotics to function, is a messy and frustrating transition.

Dance as a performance profession was perhaps not the exact path I would have followed for myself, as I gradually discovered in the unwinding of my identity. I didn't know what movement therapy was, but since my teenage years, I knew when I'd let my body move freely and turn my brain off, I felt better afterward. I was less mentally off-balance when I'd let my body play off-balance physically. Just letting myself move without any plan or structure, the body leading the way, was healing to me. Whereas dance as performance? I didn't love the perfectionism of rehearsing, nor the moments after shows where people stand around and talk. I was gifted in it though, and once you choose dance performance as your career path beyond high school, it feels like all or nothing. You can't fake it till you make it to become a professional modern dancer in the most cutthroat of all places: New York City. You have to put every ounce of your body, mind, breath, and soul into your training and networking. Every moment is a performance being judged. I had no energy for a backup plan at twenty-eight because I was excelling and feeling confident about my life. I made all my income from what I trained to do my whole life. This was something that happened to dancers in their forties or fifties, I thought. My life felt like it was slipping through my fingers. I didn't know where and when the bottom would hit.

Out of this healing crisis, I moved onto yoga and life coaching certifications, and a few years later, I began a master's program in somatic psychology. I also saw a somatic therapist. At the completion of my course studies in trauma, I broached the subject with my therapist and told her that, as a child, I was in a bad car accident and didn't know what happened.

While just talking about the trauma is not helpful by itself and can often just reinstate post-traumatic symptom cycles, being aware of the details of what happened in the event, and working with a trained somatic therapist, can help slow the symptom cycles, untangle them, and repattern in the present moment.

Close to five years after my official career transition from dance performing, I asked to speak with my parents about the accident. On a scheduled meeting, I spoke with my mother on Skype video.

"They said you would most likely grow up to have a physical disability because you broke your growth plate, which is why you got the settlement checks, I guess." She said, shrugging. "That's why they recommended you going into dance classes, for your bone health or something."

Oh, okay. Most likely grow up to have a physical disability?

Well, that was important information about *my* body for me to learn thirty years later! I was completely in shock. *You would most likely grow up to have a physical disability* was on a loop in my mind.

After the conversation, I raged. Angry, big, fat tears, sobbing for that little girl and for the grown woman who ended her dance career far too early. Moments of what felt like anxious insanity bordering on what I know to be a panic attack, and then the crash—deep depression. I texted my husband and told him we couldn't go out that right as I felt broken open. I couldn't remember the last time my nervous system exploded that way. To hold the sadness of multiple versions of myself at once was almost too much.

Before therapy and learning ways to care for myself when in distress, I don't know if I would have survived it. Unintegrated trauma in the body-mind continuum creates chronic hypo- and hyper-arousal of the nervous system. These are states that Western medicine refers to as depression and anxiety.

My thoughts were spinning into paranoia: *What is real? Do I even know my parents? Where is the ground beneath me?* I was in a trauma catharsis vortex. Too much too fast. My brain was a piece of cooked fish, my body had been fileted.

I withdraw more deeply. I didn't know how to feel about this, confused. I was numb. I entered a haze of questioning, though I knew that wouldn't help. The answers often lie in the opposite: in surrendering, releasing, and opening to a power greater than myself.

But I couldn't help it. I had entered that familiar state of analysis and preoccupation. A trauma response roughly 30 percent of Americans know well in their lifetimes, which inevitably is diagnosed as anxiety. I felt like a much younger, less safe version of myself.

Laying on the couch lifeless, I wondered: Did my parents keep this selective omission a secret all these years because they were ashamed that they had been negligent? Or did they think it would be more beneficial to ignore the possibility of pain, taking the all-too-familiar "be positive" approach?

Then I discovered more omissions. While so many of those questions remained fully unanswered and deflected, a follow-up conversation led to me asking to see the paperwork from the settlement. From these documents *I learned that the person "I" had sued for my "injuries and related lifelong suffering," and the person paying me these settlement checks was, in fact, my own father, the father I love dearly and was a safe space my entire life.* More confusion.

All these parts within me—empathy, anger, sadness, and intellectual defenses—compete for attention, for someone to hear my version of the story. It's deeply clouded my ability to be in the room, here and now. I'm frozen and dead inside and want to move this energy—yell, scream, cry, shake, something! It feels like too many unspoken stories wanting to live and breathe so badly out in the world, and out of me. I see and feel that my parents know they were in over their heads so many times. As a parent myself now, I can understand how sometimes your best just isn't enough. What if my parents were continually making decisions based on their own inherited traumas, lived traumas, and fears caused by their own PTSD?

I am stepping outside my personal pain to acknowledge the weight of intergenerational traumas I have been living out all these years. When things feel unbearable to carry alone it is because it wasn't created alone. We are the stories we have learned, we continue to tell ourselves, and we pass these onto our children in words, actions, and energy. Perhaps I can be someone to draw a line in the sand in this family, look the beast in the eye and say: no more pretending, the trauma stops here.

In my therapist's office we somatically worked with the frozen moment of impact after having learned that I was a not-buckled-in child that had flown off the seat. The body does keep the score. *Or rather, my body knew about the accident long before I did.*

This is an abbreviated version of what I went through in my session that I feel I successfully avoided for decades because of lack of information, fear, and unconscious resistance. In slow motion, we recreated where my body had blacked out: I feel my arms covering my face, my legs going limp, the lightness overcoming my body. I take a deep breath and cry. The familiar feeling of numb. Both comforting and erasing. Almost like getting high, but better—no shame involved.

"My body is so smart," I whimper and cry.

I had hated her—my body—for so long for all of this pain and confusion. It's starting to make "sense" what has happened since as a defense to the impact. Lying heavy and stuck now in a lump on my therapist's couch, but feeling that I'm in the car, turning my head, trying to see but can't, my jaw and muscles tensing. I'm hearing the screaming and trembling of my baby brother and my mother who is still in her seat. I want to reach out for my brother but can't; I want to get up but can't. My right leg feels awful.

I don't want to respond to my therapist's prompts. I feel like I'm dead, but too sad to admit it. The good news is, it's really thirty years later, and now I can. My body piecing together this narrative, but then completing the cycle of sensation and activity feels so satisfying to recreate and move the stuck traumatic energy.

"What does your body want to do now?" The therapist says. Slowly.

I want to get up and out of this car, obviously, I think. But I'm there for a long time waiting and waiting for something to shift.

Finally, I slowly start to feel my leg again and the urge to stand sets in. It's like I come back into my body, my back cracks, the little bones in my lower right leg snap, crackle, and pop. A rush of energy, I feel much taller and slowly clearer. The first breath I take in feels like I am being reborn.

"How are you now?" Fuzzy in the background. It takes a while to hear and see the room fully again. Thirty minutes have passed to express and complete what was frozen in one minute. I see my therapist so much more clearly than I ever have before. I want to hug her. But . . . I don't. I'm a little too boundless and I fear if I hugged her, I would turn into a crying baby for . . . forever. That's how deeply held I am feeling. I am relieved, and feel released, at least for now, by this powerful experience. Just one of many different somatic integrations that have kept me moving.

The goal of embodiment, it is said, is to reunite us with ourselves, bring these parts to the light. Yet, for the person with trauma, this homecoming can be painful and needs its own time to blossom. It may even be an understatement that homecoming through embodiment "can be painful;" it is some of the most difficult work to do, and humans can really be endlessly creative to avoid doing it. There are as many countless subconscious, self-sabotaging ways this happens as there are pains to be avoided. And to those who feel stuck, all over the place, and still ready to do the work, I say have faith. Liberation will eventually occur because the body wants to heal itself; the soul wants to integrate the truth.

As a dancer, I had always connected with movement therapy. I wanted and needed it like water. I had nowhere else to process pain; my parents didn't believe in therapy or God back then, so neither did I for the first half of my life. These two common places people went to seek refuge in crisis situations during my adolescent years, my core organizational system told me wouldn't work or wasn't real. I had few options, so I made my own.

When I improvised, I'd come in contact with these unintegrated fears of impact from the accident. Though they were subconsciously present all the time, in movement therapy they would rise up and take shape. There were shadow forces that would push me over, fling me sideways, or throw me down onto the floor. The gesture of hands coming up to protect my face always surfaced. These were not conscious choices (because at the time I wasn't even conscious of those memories!) but rose from the depths of my unconscious.

When given the chance to partner with another, when all five feet, ten inches of my body would be cradled and walked forward, I'd somatically remember that moment of my grandmother's sprint from the car. Every time. I can still feel the thud-thud-thud of her feet on the ground through my body, and my head resting against her racing heart. Complete surrender and love.

I am grateful for the tragedies and unique life experiences that I've come through, too. This enables me to help others. I've been able to pay for continuing education thanks to the car accident settlement check. Even before the training, it was like my soul and body knew what to do. It's been bittersweet to look back on my life's journey and see all the roads leading to here. Something was guiding me home.

Our bodies are so smart, and we can learn to access their wisdom and self-healing capacities.

"What do I do now?" I'd ask my body in moments of desperate need, paralyzed by what felt like some unbreakable mental state.

Her answer has always been, "Just keep moving."

I understand now what she was seeking because that's how trauma works. "I" was never stuck, but the memory was. Just keep moving.

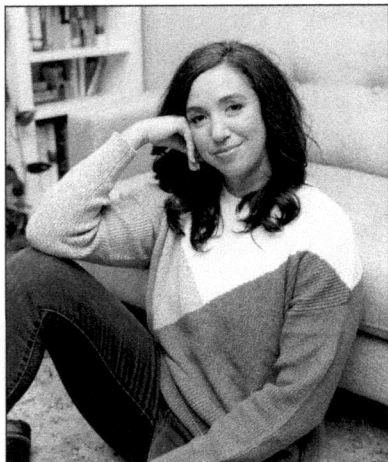

ABOUT NICOLE SMITH LEVAY

Nicole Smith Levay is an energy coach known for taking a forward-thinking and artistic approach to supporting individuals in moving beyond energetic blocks through body-centered techniques. With a background as a former professional dancer and dance teaching artist, Nicole obtained an MA in Somatic Psychology from the California Institute of Integral Studies and is a Yoga Alliance E-RYT and CEU provider, with over one thousand hours of certification. She has become a renowned workshop facilitator at esteemed healing centers such as Kripalu Center for Yoga & Health, Imiloa Institute, Ghost Ranch, and Mount Madonna Center.

One of Nicole's specialties is helping high-achieving women go from over-giving on autopilot to finally putting themselves and purpose work first. Through her company, Power Within Healing, her signature program, "Forward Momentum," and regular wellness retreats, Nicole focuses on helping individuals reclaim their energy, revive their soul work, and undergo a transformative reinvention from within. Over the past decade, a thriving community of women dedicated to living more aligned and sustainable lives has emerged around her work. Feel free to connect and become a part of this supportive network!

Follow Nicole on Facebook and Instagram @nicolesmithlevay. To book her as a speaker or workshop facilitator, please contact her directly at nicole@thepowerwithinhealing.com or (646) 926-0304.

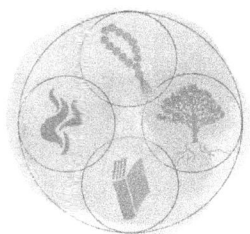

LAUGHTER AFTER TRAUMA

Deanna Salles-Freeman

As I sat in the conference listening to my mentor talk about the loss of his nephew to cancer and how he maintained gratitude through that struggle, I dug in my heels. No way was I going to be grateful for my trauma. My trauma wasn't only about me. My brother-in-law stepped in as a trusted protector after my abusive marriage ended. He introduced drugs to my kids, manipulated them, and molested my daughter. I sat in this workshop in angry tears at my vast failures as I came to the realization that I was struggling with gratitude. Gratitude—something that's supposed to be a positive force. Oh, I was grateful for the good things; that's easy, but how could I find gratitude in the worst of things? I am forever grateful for this mentor because he held me to the fire. He did not let me off the hook but told me I must find a way, my way. So, I spent the next full year doing the work. I learned so much about myself that year. I had lost my laughter. I was buried in my anger, resentment, and bitterness. I started with finding gratitude, and it came to me in the deep work I was doing on forgiveness. It was the only way through. How would I let go of this anger, resentment, and what I felt was justified indignation? I realized I was holding on to it all so that I

121

didn't have to face the real issue. I was angry at ME. I felt utterly unworthy of my relationship with my kids because I failed to protect them. I blamed myself for every bit of fallout caused by someone else's actions. This was the moment when I knew I had to forgive myself to find my laughter.

I'm naturally a lighthearted person. I love to laugh. Along the way, I realized that I had lost my fairy soul. So, I continued my rediscovery well beyond this moment that mattered. I learned that there were particular tools that allowed me to not only forgive myself but to find my laughter again. This bit of pixie dust has been my biggest blessing, and I am so happy to briefly share it. If you've ever been so hard on yourself that you feel unfit and unworthy, that deep free belly laughs are a thing of the past; then this is my gift to you. I see you. It's time for you to L.A.U.G.H.

L.A.U.G.H. is the acronym I created for the five keys to finding your laughter after trauma. Here's how it goes:

L – Let it go
A – Attitude of Gratitude
U – Undo the Negative Self-Talk
G – Give Yourself Permission
H – Heart Yourself

It took me five years to do the work that led me to this. And while there's no shortcut to healing, now you'll have the keys to unlock *your* healing journey.

Let it Go

Have you ever been consumed with something? I was in my office researching the true meaning of forgiveness. I love diving deep into the language of things in meaning and context. My first encounter with big forgiveness came when my ex-husband broke my arm. I sat in the hospital alone, abandoned by my abuser. I felt numb, void. What was wrong with *me* that I couldn't make this relationship work? There had been other incidents that left a trail that led to this sort of outcome, but I "forgave" him. I rationalized that my kids needed their father, that marriage was sacred and was forever, and that others I looked up to as examples managed to work through these things. When the marriage eventually fell apart, I decided that some things were unforgivable. My concept of forgiveness was that it condoned their horrible actions. I was not going to do that with this new trauma. I felt justified in holding onto my anger, resentment, and bitterness. But it was like holding on to the attacker and being stabbed repeatedly. What I discovered was that my suffering did not affect the perpetrator. I finally decided (yes, forgiveness is a conscious decision) to let go. I did this for me. It's a misconception that forgiveness is for others; it's always for you. Also, there are no rules. I did not feel the need to contact this person. It was a heartfelt and energetic exchange. I decided that his sick state was sad. It may well have come from abuse. I wished him healing and let go. Forgiveness allowed me to move past the wound. But something unexpected came up. I felt a lightness but not free. It was then that I discovered that I was projecting all that righteous indignation outward so that I wouldn't have to admit that I felt unforgivable. This was the biggest lesson. I approached my now-grown children and asked for forgiveness for not protecting them. They did not see it this way at all. A fantastic weight was lifted. It was here that I released the blame and guilt I was carrying. It was here that I felt free. It was here that I was able to truly *move* into gratitude.

Attitude of Gratitude

Before this whole experience, I would have said I was a grateful person. I was thankful for everything I had. I was pretty good at seeing the upside. I looked at gratitude as a scenario of "it could be worse." I called each of my kids separately. I was so scared that they would unleash years of resentment toward me. I value being a mom more than anything. I poured as much of myself as I could into creating our family. Our bond was so close that I was the one they called to hang out, go out with, ask advice, and coach through child deliveries. To possibly lose any part of that connection was terrifying, and I had avoided it by not approaching forgiveness. We had suffered some breakdown, and I wanted to heal, not just for me but for all of us. I apologized for all I felt I missed and how I failed to protect them. They expressed such love for all that I did right and no resentment for what they felt was out of my control. My connection with them is invaluable. Through all this, they have become beautifully resilient adults and parents, raising incredible little humans of their own.

Remember what I said about diving into language and context? Gratitude is not just being thankful or showing appreciation for what you have. It's not recognizing that you could be worse off—"There are starving kids in Africa." It's not rose-colored glasses and silver linings. I could not agree more with another mentor of mine, Brené Brown; gratitude is our deep appreciation for what we value, what brings meaning to our life, and what makes us feel connected to ourselves and others. I am so grateful to be on a healing adventure *along with* my children. There was much undoing that had to happen, too.

Undo the Negative Self-Talk

I had just swallowed the sleeping pill. The house was quiet. I was alone, and I needed to turn off my brain. Ever have this problem? You're falling asleep watching a show but move to the bed, and every issue from tiny to big begins playing. You spin all the ways you've messed up. So, if I wasn't out with friends, I was medicating so I could actually sleep. I had developed what I could only describe as an electrical twitch. It would jolt me straight out of my slumber. And sleep was my only escape from the voices in my head if I wasn't keeping busy. There is this constant chatter. I have it, and so do you. Always. Years of hearing how I never did the right thing, never did enough. The bills weren't paid right. The house wasn't clean enough. I didn't contribute enough to the finances. When I was alone and on my own, this soundtrack would replay on a loop. I needed a new mixed tape. Remember recording over an old cassette tape? I realized that this soundtrack had to go. Before I fell asleep that night, I said out loud to no one and everyone, "NO MORE." Mostly I said it to myself. It was a firm declaration. It was also the last night I took a sleeping aid. I began small, with affirmations and short, guided meditations. I developed my own mantra, which I repeated to myself everywhere. Out loud in the mirror first thing in the morning. As I drove around. While showering. As I drifted to sleep. Whenever a negative thought arose, I said NO and repeated my mantra. It was simple, not easy. Slowly there was a shift. This was a critical element of my healing. You must use conscious language. What we say to ourselves becomes what we believe. When the thought would come up: Jeez, you're lazy. Why do you keep procrastinating? I said, "NO! I am processing stress and taking this time for me to do so."

Here's the first mantra I created. I still say it at times. It has elevated my belief in myself tremendously.

"I am okay. I am powerful. I am more than enough. I am me, the only one, and I am beautiful and free."

Adapt mine. Make your own. Just start interrupting those negative thought patterns and flip the script.

Give Yourself Permission

I was like a zombie. About two years into the seven-year battle of my divorce, I was on the brink of breakdown. The discovery of my children's abuse and the massive action it took to have he-who-must-not-be-named arrested had kept me in "doing" mode. It had taken a toll on every aspect of my life, especially my health. Fortunately, I had an amazing support system. I hadn't noticed how much my inner circle of family and friends had stepped up. Around this time, my besties decided we needed to get away. Travel is always the answer. Renee arranged a girls' trip to EPCOT Food & Wine Fest. I was never allowed to take girls' trips in my toxic marriage. This was the first of many to come. Even though I was out of it a lot, I remember the feeling of relief. I felt like I could finally breathe. I realized on that trip that I had been "doing" non-stop for over twenty years. Bathing was my luxury, my 'me time.' I won't lie; I felt guilty about going to Disney without my kids. It seemed so wrong, and I was torn. After this trip, I knew that taking time to rejuvenate had to be non-negotiable. I wanted to give them the best of me, which was definitely not what they were getting. I used to think that self-care was a trendy phrase about pedicures and spa days. I did not understand that it meant to take care of YOURSELF, not anyone else—just you! To take the same care for yourself that you give to those you love the most was a profound lesson. I had never taken care of myself to that level. Sometimes I still don't. I will forever be a work in progress.

Heart Yourself

Like self-care, self-love has become a buzzword. It has lost its meaning in its overuse and misuse. I was staring at myself in the mirror. It was the second day of a 21-day mirror work challenge I had taken on. I looked at myself as instructed, and using my name, I attempted to say, "Deanna, I love you. I really, really love you." Except, it came out choked. My body was tense and a little shaky. Then, the tears began to roll. All I could think was that I felt like I was in the right place for myself and that I was also a disappointment to some people who mattered to me the most. I could not reconcile it. I'd always done what was expected of me. Often it still was not enough. I was emerging in a spiritual sense, and it did not fully align with my upbringing. I felt a deep spiritual connection, yet I also felt I wasn't doing what I "should" be doing. What did I do? Turned to travel, of course. There is nothing like nature to help you get grounded and connected to yourself and to something greater than yourself. What better place than a place rooted in spirituality? Hawaii. I made myself a promise to be present—leave all the expectations, guilt, and shame behind. I even extended my stay a week to ensure I could immerse myself in nature and exploration. I rented a Jeep. As I drove out on the first day, I reached the top of a mountain road and looked out. I was immediately overcome with tears. I had to stop for a second. There was a lava field to my right, black and barren. You could see and feel what the movement had been, slow and wavy. To my left was a grassy field with goats grazing—land that was alive. Forward was the most picturesque view I had ever seen. It was a pristine beach with these perfect trees, their trunks twisted, and their branches umbrellaed into the perfect shade. Beyond that was crystal clear water, a gradient from aqua to deep blue. I sat and just breathed. I am okay. It is okay to be me. Just as I am, right here and right now. I was growing and changing. I loved what I was becoming, and, at this moment, I accepted myself for who I was. That's self-love. This is how you "heart yourself."

The Laughter After

There is such freedom in being okay with being yourself. The weight I had carried trying to do and be what was expected was slowly lifting. I started to get back to that fun-loving little girl, my fairy soul. She is light and comfortable just being herself. On a girls' trip to EPCOT Food & Wine Fest some years later, we found ourselves following the 80s love ballad band Air Supply. On one particular day, we set out to catch all three shows they were doing. In between, we had a passport to fill with various food and libations. By the second show, I was feeling good, maybe even a little too good. One of our friends is reliant on a wheelchair. We were heading back for the last show, but a bathroom break was urgently needed. We stopped at the family restroom, which was also equipped for handicapped use. I helped her onto the toilet and realized that I had to go too bad to be able to lift her off. It was a dilemma. We began to laugh, which didn't help matters. My friend then dared me to use the urinal in the family-equipped bathroom. I took this as a challenge and readily accepted it. Hold my phone. As I extended my backside way out and hovered masterfully, I began to relieve myself. At this point, my friend was so impressed she decided to capture a picture. Unwittingly, she held the camera button and captured twenty-seven pictures. We finished up, laughing so much that the others needed to know what was so funny. I showed them. Don't worry; I just looked bent over with my hands on my knees. We went to our concert. Sang our hearts out. As we left, I got a group chat message from the man that would become my husband. We were dating, and he was saying good night. Another dare came in to show him how talented I am at hovering. In my feel-good state, I sent all twenty-seven pictures. My sisters were also in this chat, one of whom politely told me this was not sexy. We stopped for pizza on the boardwalk and laughed at my expense until I hurt. I was still sore the next day. I hadn't realized that I hadn't let go and hadn't just been myself until this moment. This was the moment I knew I had found my laughter after trauma.

I see you, and you are beautiful!

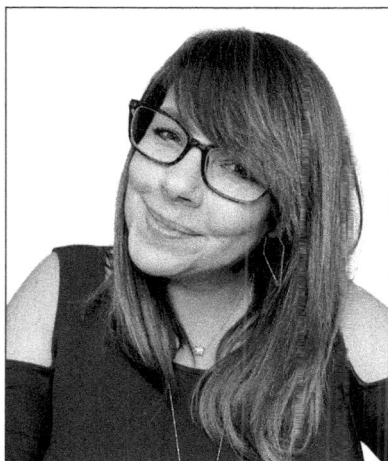

ABOUT DEANNA SALLES-FREEMAN

Deanna is a speaker, author, and highly certified coach in multiple disciplines, bringing light and lightness to the heavy topic of trauma. Her personal journey with intimate partner violence (IPV) and as a parent of survivors has led her to find beauty and laughter in healing. Today, Deanna has dedicated her life to helping moms break free from guilt and find THEIR laughter after. She specializes in creating unique keynotes and workshops for women's retreats. She has partnered with Oola™ as a mentor coach and incorporates the lifestyle system that initiated her transformation into her personalized programs.

Go to my website to book a free discovery call.

https://deannawellness.com
Instagram: https://instagram.com/deannawellness
Facebook: https://facebook.com/deannawellness
LinkedIn: https://www.linkedin.com/in/deanna-salles-freeman
Threads: https://threads.net/@deannawellness
Podcast: *Laughter After Trauma* on all major podcast platforms
Apple: https://podcasts.apple.com/us/podcast/laughter-after-trauma/id1632469554

To get weekly inspiration every Monday straight to your phone, text the word 'loop' to 985-205-8484.

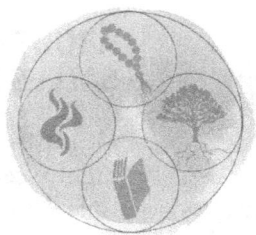

GRATITUDE IN TIMES OF DESPAIR: PARADOXES FOR WHOLENESS

Ericha Scott, PhD

t is easy to feel gratitude or thankfulness when life circum-stances go our way. It is fun to celebrate, for example, a new job or a promotion, a new or rekindled romance, financial wind-falls, graduations, or retirement—and recognition for our natural talents or hard work.

It is much more difficult to feel gratitude when we are chal-lenged with relational strife, grief and loss, trauma, abuse, addic-tion, illness, poverty, or alienation.

I have learned about the power of gratitude by watching my clients.

I have worked with clients who were nearly destroyed by abuse, trauma, and sometimes even systematic and sophisticated torture—and yet, they found a moment or moments of gratitude.

They found these moments in the midst of a history of horror and the aftermath.

Observing that first moment, the dawning of thankfulness, is as wondrous as watching birth, and in fact, it is a birth of a spiri-tual life. Watching a client's face as it shifts and changes with the new awareness that life is precious is to bear witness to profound beauty.

Survivors of trauma, mental illness, and addiction have taught me the true meaning of thankfulness and gratitude.

Gratitude can be triggered by a small find in nature, a loving comment by a friend, a thoughtful gift, a break from suffering, an observation of selflessness in another, or the claiming of a talent. This form of gratitude is more often born from a small event of low monetary value than from a new car or TV.

We can all learn from those who have been shattered by grief and their determination to recover. It might sound superficial, but I have thought, *If they can do it, so can I.*

Scientific research supports my clinical observations regarding the positive impact of gratitude and thankfulness on physical and mental health. Although not all research is equal, many studies reveal a variety of significant benefits such as improved:

1. relationships

2. physical health and sleep

3. mental health and happiness

4. empathy for others

5. resilience from trauma

6. self-esteem

For many people, especially survivors of addiction and trauma, feelings of gratitude do not come naturally. Therefore, I encourage my clients to develop a daily practice of gratefulness, even if it feels fake at first. This practice is a disciplined approach versus an organic one. An example of a simple disciplined practice is one suggested by Salt Lake City therapist Debbie Reid, CSW, during our telephone call. She suggests to "write down two things each day for which I am thankful." She also suggests "writing down five ways I can show gratitude to others during the day." Those in a twelve-step program know that people with addiction who are newly sober are often asked by old timers to be grateful even if it's just for "a roof over my head, food on my plate, and shoes on my feet." It seems as if gratitude magnifies abundance.

All of my life I have struggled with negativity. Even as a very small child, I remember snuggling next to my mother in bed as she read out loud, *The Little Engine That Could*, by Watty Piper. It was her wish that the story of the kind, blue engine might inspire me to try and succeed in kindergarten. This story illustrates how well I know the difficulty of feeling grateful when negative thoughts cloud your mind.

In the following paragraphs, I will offer a few healing directives and activities. Hopefully, you will find these exercises compelling and attractive. I know from experience they are effective. If you have any doubts about an activity, please take this chapter to a mentor or your therapist and ask if you should try these suggestions. This is a great way to take care of yourself while strengthening your recovery.

The best intervention for negative thoughts I have learned was taught to me by author Pia Melody almost forty years ago. Her directives were not simple or easy, but I found them to be very powerful. Her guidance fostered one of my first steps toward wholeness.

Pia asked me to write down twenty negative thoughts about myself. I ask people to do this and to also include negative thoughts, or generalizations, about their perceptions of the world as it is. I recommend dividing your journal paper into two vertical columns. List the negative beliefs on the left, then positively reframe each one on the right.

Writing these negative thoughts and positive affirmations down empower and anchor the exercise, versus just thinking or talking about them. In other words, the outcome of your personal work is likely to be more effective.

For example, I find it difficult to organize my office desk. Therefore, on the left column, I might write, "I am disorganized." I can reframe this sabotaging belief by writing the exact opposite statement in the right column, even if it is not true yet: "I am organized." This type of simple reframe works fine.

I can strengthen the comment, "I am organized" by adding a few facts that contradict my negative belief system. This type of statement might be, "I hired the help I need to straighten up my desk and office," "I organized my desk and office space, so my life is more efficient, and I have fewer distractions," or "It is not an accident I have a doctorate and published research." If you are not able to be as direct with your reframes as the examples above, then consider starting each positive affirmation statement with, "I am able to organize my desk."

Your subconscious only needs for you to be open to the possibilities for healing. It is like cracking open a small window in a large room, just a little bit to freshen up the stagnant odor. It always surprises me how well it works.

After I have written at least twenty positive statements, all written as "I" statements, I follow up several ways. One activity I use is to make a recording of the self-loving, positive comments, in my own voice. I listen to these digital recordings when my confidence is wavering, or my negativity has peaked. One time, as I listened to my own voice, I realized I had written a very personal type of prose poem, like the "Desiderata" (things desired), a poem written by Max Ehrmann in the 1920s.

It is most effective to listen to your recording in your voice on a daily basis. It is okay to listen to your affirmations and gratitude list almost any time or place you want, so long as it is safe. You might listen to your personal Desiderata while cooking, or on the patio watching a sunset, or during a lunch break at work. It is even more powerful to listen to these recordings while looking into your own eyes in a mirror.

Recording our self-loving prose is much easier to do today than forty years ago now that we have audio and video recorders on our phones and computers.

I make my own greeting cards, and I use them often to write

notes of appreciation and gratitude to those I love. I know this might sound amusing, but I feel as if I have added a "spiritual sweetener" to some of my relationships with close friends and social connections, even those that were a little bit challenging. People are better able to receive and believe notes of love when they read them in your own handwriting.

It is important for counselors and therapists to note even the simple exercise of writing an affirmation or gratitude list can trigger protests from clients, as if one positive word or action invalidates decades of pain. Positive words and actions do not invalidate past suffering. Although, and this may seem ironic, it is true that positive words can trigger unconscious grief or the unexpressed pain of times when a person's suffering was minimized or invalidated.

As a coach, counselor, or therapist, it is important to be very sensitive to this dynamic. It can be helpful to predict in advance, that for some people, affirmations of life can bring up unidentified grief, shame, and anger. This reaction should be described to the client as normative and a short, small, temporary step in the process of positive change.

One potent way to process the inner negative responses to positive list-making is to write down the negative thoughts or rebuttals as they emerge. Very simply, list the gratitude items on your paper and the negative responses below, then write the positive statement again, and repeat until the negative thoughts have dissipated a little bit or completely. This process might feel great, and yet you may want to share your list with a therapist or a safe mentor. This way, the negative beliefs can be evaluated for possible dysfunctional family or cultural myths or lies.

In my own healing process, one of the issues I have addressed with positive words and paintings of gratitude is my creative intelligence. As a child, I was considered to be "retarded," when in fact, I was gifted. This falsehood outlasted evidence to the contrary. For example, after I graduated with a master's degree and a GPA of 3.94 (out of 4.0), I had to make a conscious choice to honor my intelligence, even though I had received concrete validation. Trusting my creative intelligence did not come naturally. The familial messages carried weight long-term.

The practice of gratitude for my strengths, even before I was able to see them clearly, helped me take good care of myself and push beyond limited and sabotaging negative parental expectations.

It is important to include a note of caution here. There can be a dark side to the practice of gratitude and affirmations, especially when it is not grounded in stability, sobriety, or reality. This might be completely surprising in an era of positive psychology; yet there is a risk of using gratitude and affirmations to feed denial or reinforce unhealthy behaviors. For example, most people who are chemically dependent, at some point, felt very grateful for the relief or high their use provided. Yet, to dwell on that specific moment—the minute of relief—after a shot of hard liquor, a needle prick of the skin, a snort of powder or smoke, or the swallowing of a handful of pills without also noting the perils of addiction can be very destructive.

This type of ungrounded positivity helps us deny or postpone our pain, which can seem like a good thing, but it keeps us stuck. The challenge is to write a gratitude or affirmation list that stretches us beyond our false limitations, yet remains healthy, sustainable, and realistic.

In addition, for those with a serious mental illness, especially with delusions or grandiosity, a therapist's assignment should be tailored to the specific needs of the client. It is important to be sure that grandiosity and delusions are not amplified or reinforced.

Robert Fritz, a theorist who writes about creativity in *The Path of Least Resistance*, offers a complementary practice to gratitude and affirmations.

He boldly says that NO GOAL is too big to create! Robert says that to create a goal, it is essential to be grounded in the current reality that is pertinent to the dream you want to manifest in the future. Basically, he is saying, dream big but know where you are. He suggests, in a way that is not that different from Carl Jung's mandala polarities, to juxtapose the vision you want to create right alongside the reality of what you have and don't have. In other words, it is essential to hold or juxtaposition the polarity of the opposites, images of where you are now and where you want to go. It does not matter how large the differential between the two. To hold the polarities, I use list-making, charts, collages, mandalas, and paintings.

Just think, even the atoms in our cells have a form of negative and positive structural tension. The best way to make tension productive is to channel it into creativity.

It is the "structural tension" between two polarities or opposites, and how it engages and includes your subconscious mind, that helps spark creative ideas and concrete manifestations. This is like a flint being scraped against carbon steel to create a fire. This process works—often in tandem with other activities—for psychological, emotional, spiritual, cognitive, and physical health. At one point, when I had a physical challenge, I painted in a mandala my version of healthy cells, copied from the encyclopedia, and my own cells, which were not as healthy as I would have liked, copied from images made by a dark field microscope. This was one of many integrative medicine or alternative interventions I used when I had cancer. With a wide range of interventions, I was able to overcome this serious and potentially fatal problem.

I know it seems as if I am repeating myself, but it took me a while to fully grasp this concept. Creativity arises out of the tension between spontaneity and limitations, the latter (like riverbanks directing the flow of a river) forcing the spontaneity into the various forms that are essential to a work of literature, art, music, dance, theater, or film.

Personally, I feel the most gratitude when I am immersed in a creative flow, especially when I am accurately portraying my inner world! Catharsis, or release, happens when a person is portraying an accurate symbol of their inner experience. This is one reason the creative arts are such a good modality for people in pain or struggling with compulsions.

For a long time, I have been asking clients to look at the visual art they have made about the polarities of their lives and breathe in the whole art piece, not just the happy, positive portion. One of the first times I asked a client to do this, there was a lot of darkness and self-hate on the large painting. Reluctantly, she did as I asked and said, "For the first time in my life, I am ALL here! I have insides, they are mine, and I am not giving them away!"

Recently a client expressed fear about breathing in the dark and the light of her painting. She said, "I am afraid that the dark blob of paint that looks like a monster will hurt me." I responded with, "It is already hurting you." Almost immediately after breathing in the whole polarity she said, "I feel much stronger. I hear the word no. I feel as if I need to say no more often."

Once a student made a mask of her self-hate. It was even hard for me to look at and I am used to looking at heavy material. At the end of our training, I found her cradling her mask in her arms, rocking it like a beloved baby. She beamed up at me with an enormous smile and said, "My self-hate had trapped my power!" The integrity of her mask painting was liberating for her. She felt power, joy, and gratitude.

For me, it has been a long tango-type of dance toward gratitude with many missteps. This dance included the dark and the light, passion, intensity, quiet and silent still moments, poems, paintings, sculptures, list making, affirmations, gratitude lists, and more. None of this work would have been successful without authentic and honest truth telling—and some of that was ugly. So yes, make your affirmation and gratitude lists, but please do not stop there because there is so much more wholeness waiting for you to be had with the stroke of a crayon, brush, or pen.

Again, performing the simplest healing actions, over and

over, ultimately take us where we need to go. Along with written affirmations, gratitude lists, recordings, paintings, and "breathing in the polarities" as mentioned above, these practices will aid you on your path to wholeness. Your way is the right way, and I trust you will find which activities to include on your unique creative journey.

In these challenging times, it is important to include this note of caution. Mental health and addiction problems have been on the rise since the beginning of the pandemic. The increase in anxiety, substance use disorders, and depression linger even now that the pandemic is no longer considered a direct threat. If you find that therapy and the exercises included in this chapter are not sufficient to reduce your despair, please do not delay and call the National Suicide and Crisis Hotline 988. Please call as many times as you need. Your life matters.

In summary, if you need more gratitude in your life, the exercises in this chapter will help you. If the suggestions mentioned above seem overwhelming, then please consider starting with something easier like mindfulness walks and focus on the beauty of nature. Pick up found objects and look at them carefully, allow yourself to feel a bit of curiosity, awe, and wonder. Other suggestions for adding more gratitude and positivity to your life include dancing, writing poetry, making music, filming a video, writing an autobiography, or painting and sculpting. You might ask a friend to share bidirectionally, even if only by text, thankful and grateful thoughts. Please interview your friends about what they appreciate and find meaningful about their lives and about you. I recommend art, intuitive dance, music, and poetry making parties on the theme of gratitude in times of despair. Consider adding thanksgiving to your time in prayer and meditation, and finally, you could be especially courageous and speak of your gratitude directly to and for the loved ones in your life such as family, friends and even colleagues. Of course, you could hand-write a good old fashioned love letter to yourself or someone else.

These practices of appreciation, affirmations, love and gratitude, no matter how small, if practiced consistently, gather depth and breadth over time.

Many people include gratitude as part of their spiritual practice. Again, it is also used by people who want to improve their mood, health, sleep, and relationships. Gratitude does not mean you have to be fake.

Gratitude gives people hope and the strength to endure. It can sustain and inspire us during times of personal, community and global despair. Simply said, gratitude is a very powerful healing tool.

It is my wish everyone will have moments of genuine and wholesome gratitude in their lives.

"Gratitude bestows reverence, allowing us to encounter everyday epiphanies, those transcendent moments of awe that change forever how we experience life and the world."

—John Milton

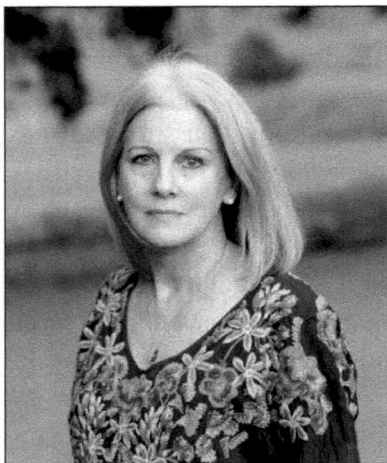

ABOUT ERICHA SCOTT, PHD, LPCC917, ICAADC, ICRC, ATR-BC, REAT

For thirty-eight years, Dr. Scott has been a healer who walks the fine line between mysticism and evidenced-based psychotherapy.

She is a Licensed Clinical Professional Counselor (LPCC917) in California. She has been initiated in several shamanic traditions, certified as an interfaith spiritual director, energy healer, advanced substance use disorder counselor, and she is a dually certified creative and expressive arts therapist. She is a keynote speaker, and she has contributed to several collaborative books ranked as #1 international best sellers. She paints, takes photographs, and writes poetry.

She has designed and facilitated numerous art psychoeducational and creative arts therapeutic workshops and has been recognized throughout the United States and abroad for her original, unique, and powerful healing experiences. Recently, she presented for the first scientific creative arts therapy conference in the Middle East for the Egyptian Art Therapy Association in Cairo, Egypt.

Dr. Scott is accepting clients for two-to-five-day private, individual, and custom-designed creative arts intensives in Malibu. These intensives include Jungian sand play therapy, painting, self-portraits, life-sized silhouette mandalas (body maps), abstract murals, sculpture, art in nature (eco-psychology), drumming, therapeutic writing, poetry, role play, and more. If you want to expand your consciousness and your life, please call Dr. Ericha Scott.

To Connect with Dr. Scott

www.artspeaksoutloud.org

To book her as a speaker, retreat leader, or for creative and expressive arts intensives in her studio office, please contact her directly at 310-880-9761.

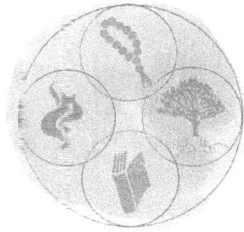

THE MOMENT OF DECISION

Elie D. Shefi

"It is in the moments of decision that your destiny is shaped."

—Tony Robbins

Right or left?
Stay or go?
Do I or don't I?

Crossroads. We've all stood at them, that fork where different paths converge and we must make a choice. We've all faced tough decisions and made choices that changed our lives.

Decisions are so difficult because they are powerful. They matter. They have the power to uproot our lives. And the power to maintain the status quo. Are you mindful of your decisions? Do you make them consciously and intentionally? Or are you living life on autopilot, just getting through each day?

I lived on autopilot for years. I behaved the way others expected. I did what they demanded. I even mindlessly ate what they placed before me. I made no conscious decisions, and I lived a robotic life utterly void of authenticity, abundance, and joy.

I relinquished all control of my life and let my circumstances dictate my existence. You see, I'm an abuse survivor, rape survivor, and domestic violence survivor who has lived in hiding under a fake name. I've struggled financially, lived in my car, and asked restaurants for the food they were throwing away at the end of the night. I'm a cancer survivor and medical miracle who has had thirteen major surgeries and has been defying the doctors' death deadlines for more than twenty years.

And yet, despite those events and circumstances, I've learned to take back control over my life, make intentional decisions, harness my power, and create a life I love! I may have been forged by fire, but I am free by design.

Through almost five decades of getting back up every time life has knocked me down, I've learned to live life on my terms and decide who I want to be and how I want to show up in the world. Now I unapologetically stand in my power and use my voice to empower others. I'm an attorney, advisor, advocate, coach, consultant, speaker, strategist, #1 International Best-selling and award-winning author, publisher, philanthropist, podcast and TV host, the discrimination and human rights lawyer of the year, a New York Times power lawyer, one of the most influential women leaders to watch, one of the most admired women leaders in business, and one of the top entrepreneurs changing the game in 2023.

How did I make such drastic changes? Through moments of decision. Everything changed for me when I began making conscious decisions—when I took control of my path, my destiny, my business, my health, my relationships, my life!

While all moments matter, the moments of decision are the moments that will change and shape your life. You see, your decisions fuel your actions. And it's your actions that fuel your clarity and your path forward.

In those moments of decision—those moments when you draw a line in the sand and decide that something has to change, something needs to be different—you start to take action. At that first moment, you probably won't be clear on the whole path, and you won't have all the details. But because you've made the decision, you're able to take one step, one action, which then leads to another step, another action, and then the path will unfold. Clarity comes from action.

We can live a life by design when we consciously and intentionally choose our decisions as they are the foundation upon which an authentic, free life is built.

I've had four key moments of decision in my life.

Choosing Me

I'm a domestic violence survivor. I was friends with my ex-husband for years before we married, but the person he admired as a friend was anathema to who he needed as a spouse. He tried to mold me into his ideal wife through whatever means necessary. I initially stayed in the marriage so as to not have to face my own mother's ridicule (she had placed bets with her family on how long the marriage would last). And, over time, I was broken down to merely following the path of least resistance. *If I just do what I'm told, then maybe I won't get hurt.* That was my life for two years. In my mind, the path of least resistance equaled survival. But it actually meant my death.

Things got bad during the summer of 2000. I was supposed to be starting my second year of law school, but instead, I was in the hospital from the stress of living in fight-or-flight—my organs and bodily systems were failing. I had developed somatoform disorder. My body physically manifested my emotional trauma. A doctor who figured out that spousal abuse was causing my illness contacted my father and said, "I think this is what's happening, and your daughter will be dead by Christmas."

Well, that was all my father needed to hear. He reached out to the local law enforcement, and he organized my rescue. I had no part in the plan. I knew the situation was dire, but I would not leave on my own. I was so debilitated that I was a shell, an automaton that simply did what I was told by my ex-husband. My health had deteriorated to the extent that my life literally depended on the help of others to get me out. Four police officers plus my dad came to our apartment. Two officers pinned down my ex-husband while two took my arms and pulled me out. My dad waited in a running car, and as soon as the officers put me in the back seat, he hit the gas and drove thirty-eight hours across the country to get me to safety.

I was put into hiding and given a fake name. I became a ghost—on paper and to myself. I was placed in a home with a man I didn't know. I was terrified and would barricade the doors and windows. I barely left my room and had lost all ability to make a decision. Every single day for months, I ate the exact same thing for breakfast, lunch, and dinner because no one told me what to eat, and I was not capable of making my own decisions or functioning independently.

I spent hours each day, month after month, in intense trauma therapy. One day, my therapist challenged me to go to the grocery store on my own. My assignment was simply to buy something—anything—from the store. I couldn't do it. I ran out of the store in tears, hysterical because I couldn't even decide what to buy. As I stood in the grocery store parking lot, sobbing uncontrollably and utterly broken, something shifted in me. That's when I had my first major moment of decision. I finally understood that, if things were going to get better, I had to make a choice.

I had to be the one to decide that my life was worth more, that I was worth more. I had to be the one to decide that I was worth living a joyful life I loved.

Instead of seeing myself as the girl whose future had been snatched from her, I had to choose to see my situation as an opportunity. "I am complete ashes," I told myself. "This is ground zero for my life. What an incredible opportunity I have to start over from scratch and rebuild myself into exactly who I want to be. What an amazing gift that, in starting over, I get to define for myself who I will be, what I will stand for, and how I will live my life from this point forward. What freedom!"

I recognized right then and there that my experiences were a blessing. I finally understood that I was powerful beyond measure, and that I actually had control over my life in all aspects—even those that I had thus far felt powerless to control. I realized that I had the power to write my own story the way I wanted it to be . . . not my ex-husband, not my parents, not society, and not labels placed on me by an outside observer. *Me.* I had the power to choose. And I had the power to do and be anyone and anything I desired. I had the power to create and live life on my own terms.

A lot has happened in the decades since my rescue and resurrection. I've continued to design my life deliberately and with intention, based on that initial moment of decision, through every obstacle life has thrown my way. Just because I decided to take control of my life once, however, doesn't mean that I'm magically in this impervious, unshakable state of perpetual power and positivity. Choosing how I show up in each moment is a daily decision, a daily practice.

But, by doing this every single day, external circumstances no longer define me. The views of others no longer define me. I define myself.

Choosing My Future

I spent a year away from law school healing and rebuilding my life. After about five months in hiding, I moved to Europe. While there, I met five incredible women who became my sisters, and through their love, patience, compassion, and support, I came back to life. The love of this sisterhood healed me, and I built the new me from ashes. It also was the catalyst for much of the work that I do now with women, like my Sedona Sisterhood Retreats, my Sisters Rising book series, and my individual coaching, to help guide them to rise up, claim their voices, and step into their power!

My life in Europe was good, and I was happy. I had learned

how to function independently again. I was living, I was laughing, and I was thriving.

But, according to the rules of the American Bar Association, a student had to spend at least two of their three years of law school in residence at the degree-granting institution in order to receive their Juris Doctorate from that institution, and they had to graduate within five years of matriculating. So there came a moment when I had to decide whether to come out of hiding and finish law school so I could graduate within the permissible timeframe, or whether to remain safely and happily in Europe with my support system.

This second major moment of decision—of facing fear and choosing me . . . of staring down my past and choosing my future—was not an easy one.

Ultimately, I decided that my ex-husband had already taken enough from me. I decided that while he had broken my spirit, taken my very identity, and caused my body to shut down, I would not let him take anything else from me. I refused to let him take my dreams or my future, so I chose me, and I chose to return to law school. However, my ex-husband was still in the vicinity.

Choosing Gratitude

I got my law degree—my ticket to my future—but at the cost of my health. The stress of my ex-husband being nearby and following me and trying to contact me caused me to live that year in perpetual fight-or-flight mode and caused prolonged trauma exposure. I got sick again. So very, very sick. I was diagnosed with adrenal tumor Cushing's syndrome and had the first few of what would be thirteen major surgeries.

From that point, I spent the better part of two decades living in and out of hospitals, fighting for my life. By 2007, I had grown tired of the pain, tired of the struggle, and tired of the constant fight to survive. I was giving up. I had had enough. I was done fighting the doctors' death deadlines. Then one day, everything changed. It was a day I had to have another excruciating test. When it was time for me to go for testing, the porter came to get me from my room and wheeled my wheelchair down hallways that he had never taken me through before.

He wheeled me through the hallways of the area in the hospital where everyone was on a ventilator, either paralyzed from the neck down or in a coma. I looked into room after room and realized that any one of those patients would give anything to feel the pain I was feeling. In an instant, I realized that my pain was an incredible blessing and that I was so lucky to be able to feel it travel around my body. I thanked God that I still had nerves that were connected and synapses that were firing as they should. What a gift! I turned my pity party into gratitude, and my weariness became resolve. I was flooded with gratitude for my body and all it provided me.

In that third major moment of decision, I once again took control of my life; this time by embracing the power of gratitude.

Have you ever noticed that when you allow yourself to feel truly grateful about something, you cannot simultaneously feel angry, anxious, fearful, worried, or frustrated?

Go ahead—try it. Think of something for which you are truly and deeply grateful. Put yourself back in that beautiful moment. Notice how you feel. Notice the warmth. Notice the sense of peace. Notice the love. Notice the joy. Notice the appreciation. Of course, you can feel anger, worry, fear, or frustration before and after you feel grateful, but negative emotions are impossible to feel at the same time as gratitude.

Feeling grateful interrupts whatever negative emotion you're experiencing long enough to help you shift your perspective and fuel your strength to persevere.

The ability to find and feel true gratitude is the ultimate mind hack. It is a powerful tool—one that can be learned. On the days when you feel like the walls are caving in, use gratitude as the hook to pull you to safety. In the moments when you are weary and feel like you just can't go on, find something in your life to be grateful for. Something . . . anything. It's there! Give thanks for the breath you take, the roof over your head, the bed that you sleep in, the blanket that keeps you warm. Give thanks for the senses you have, for the electricity you have, for the running water you have, for the food you eat. Seek your blessings and feel grateful. Now, living in gratitude takes some practice, but the more you practice, the stronger it will be.

Choosing Authenticity and Stepping Into My Power

Despite all the sickness and surgeries, once I received my law degree, I did build a life that I loved—a life I promised myself in that grocery store parking lot!

I moved to Nashville and began my work as a staff attorney for a federal judge. It's incredibly meaningful work. As a staff attorney, I am the right hand of the judge on the bench. A judge has hundreds of cases at a time, and it's the staff attorney who reads them, looks at every piece of evidence, and analyzes and determines how the law applies. The judge gets the final say, but I provide the research and the legal advice. In this, I've dedicated my life to giving a voice to the voiceless, to seeing people, to hearing people, to making sure every single word that they write to the court is considered.

And if they've met the requirements of the law, they win; if they don't, they lose. But I write a court decision where they know that they were seen, they were heard, and their voice mattered. The bulk of my work is employment and education discrimination and prison condition cases, but I do handle all constitutional claims and civil rights violations. When I began this stage of my career, I was able to successfully build my life where I could have the impact I wanted and use my voice. But in a way that felt safe, protected.

And then, in January 2019, I found out I had uterine cancer. After nineteen years of fighting for my life, surviving surgery after surgery after surgery, and being a medical miracle, I heard the words that no one wants to hear: "Ellie, we have your pathology reports, and I'm sorry, but it's cancer." Time stopped.

It was time for my fourth major moment of decision. What would I do?

In that moment of deafening silence, I said to myself, *I've been playing small.* And I decided, *No more. Now is the time.* You see, I had built this comfortable, impact-driven bubble where I had been able to work behind the scenes. I'd been content to be the advisor or the anonymous donor. But right then and there, everything changed. I made a promise to myself: *I don't know how much time I have, but I know this: I'm stepping out of the shadows, and I am stepping up my impact to a global scale. I will impact lives every day that I have left on this planet.* My life became clear at that moment.

I stopped hiding behind the curtain. I stepped out front and really stepped into my own voice, into my own purpose, and into my own power. And from that moment on, I have truly lived the life that I was meant to live.

Choosing Every Moment

"You are one decision away from a completely different life."

—Mel Robbins

These four moments of decision have shaped my life by guiding me to clarity—to my why, my passions, my mission, and my purpose. This clarity acts as both my fuel and my anchor. It gives me the strength to get up and the fuel to persist, while allowing me to remain focused and grounded. I know that I was made to change the world. It's my mission and purpose to ignite impact, empower transformation, and facilitate change on a global scale. Because my why, my mission, and my purpose are bigger than me, they allow me to focus on serving others, which allows me to get out of my own way, choose conviction over convenience, and remain resilient, unbreakable, and unstoppable.

Your moments of decision are waiting for you. You just have to be open to them. You don't have to be at ground zero or completely reduced to ashes to grasp them. You don't need to wait for drama or catastrophe. Every moment is an opportunity to decide whether you're staying in the status quo or whether it's time for a change. What will you choose?

Remember, you're always one decision away from the rest of your life. Choose wisely. Make every moment matter.

Because you matter.

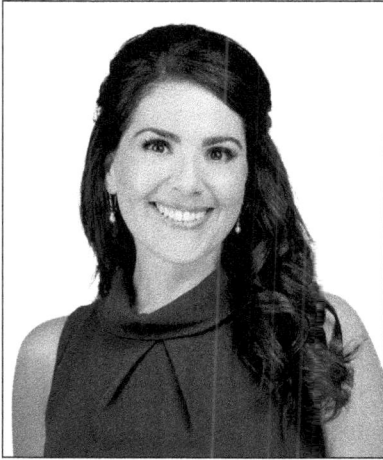

ABOUT ELLIE D. SHEFI

Ellie Shefi is an attorney, advisor, leadership consultant, corporate trainer, keynote speaker, strategist, and #1 International Best-selling and award-winning author who helps organizations optimize their culture and individuals expand their influence.

As the founder of MTC Consulting, Ellie leverages her more than thirty years of experience in law, business, education, and advocacy to help organizations build resilient teams and world-class cultures while developing influential leaders. Serving as a strategic advisor to governments, universities, corporations, entrepreneurs, and NGOs, she has successfully helped organizations mitigate their risk, optimize their operations, and align their teams.

Dedicated to empowering others to use their voice, Ellie founded Made to Change the World Publishing, a full-service independent publishing house, where she guides aspiring best-selling authors through the writing and publishing process and helps leaders amplify their message so they can scale their impact.

A sought-after keynote speaker, Ellie is regularly interviewed in top publications and on podcasts and media channels like *Forbes*, *Entrepreneur*, NBC, ABC, and CBS, among others, and she hosts the *Free by Design* television show, the *Creating an Impervious Mind*® YouTube series, and the *You Are Not Your Scars*® podcast.

Ellie is also the founder of the Made 2 Change the World Foundation, an emerging nonprofit organization that equips and empowers the next generation with the tools, resources, and strategies they need to create the lives, communities, and world they envision.

To connect with Ellie, please visit:

www.ellieshefi.com

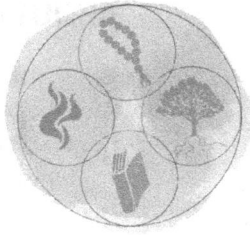

Have you ever of
becoming a published author?
Do you have a story to share?
Would the world benefit
from hearing your message?

Then we want to connect with you!

The *Inspired Impact Book Series* is looking to connect with women who desire to share their stories with the goal of inspiring others.

We want to hear your story!

Visit www.katebutlerbooks.com to learn more about becoming a Featured Author in the #1 International Best-selling *Inspired Impact Book Series.*

Everyone has a story to share!
Is it your time to create your legacy?

inspired **IMPACT**
BOOK SERIES

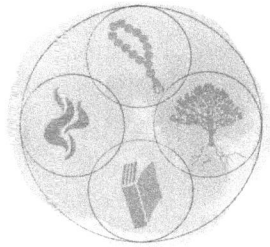

May your soul be uplifted and the words of these pages inspire you to continue to lead with your infinite divine light to your fullest expression in leaving your legacy!

Authors of Moments That Matter

REPRINTED WITH PERMISSIONS

Eichelle V. Thompson
Patty Aubery
Kate Butler, CPSC
Bella Butler
Erin Saxton
Jenna Edwards
Marisa Griffin
Erica Rasmussen
Tiffany Donovan Green
Danielle Lynn
Danny W. Pettry II
Michelle Picking
Amber Whitt
Tracey Watts Cirino
Alexia Clonda
Jennifer Eaker
Ann Marie Gill
Nicole Smith Levay
Deanna Salles-Freeman
Ericha Scott, PhD
Ellie D. Shefi